Aromatherapy for the
Healthy Child

Aromatherapy for the
Healthy Child

more than 300 natural, nontoxic, and fragrant essential oil blends

VALERIE ANN WORWOOD

New World Library
Novato, California

New World Library
14 Pamaron Way
Novato, CA 94949

Copyright © 2000 by Valerie Ann Worwood
Cover photograph: Kathryn Kleinman
Cover and text design: Mary Ann Casler

The material in this book is not meant to take the place of diagnosis and treatment by a qualified medical practitioner. All recommendations herein contained are believed to be effective, but since actual use of essential oils by others is beyond the author's or publisher's control, no expressed or implied guarantee as to the effects of their use can be given nor liability taken. Any application of the recommendations set forth in the following pages is at the reader's sole risk. Essential oils are to be used at the reader's sole risk and at the reader's own discretion.

Most of the suggestions and recipes outlined in this book can be used alongside most modern day pharmaceuticals and as a first aid measure. It is suggested that you consult your pediatrician/physician with full details of what you wish to use before doing so.

Library of Congress Cataloging-in-Publication Data
Worwood, Valerie Ann, 1945–
     Aromatherapy for the healthy child : more than 300 natural, nontoxic, and fragrant essential oil blends / Valerie Ann Worwood.
        p.   cm
        Includes bibliographical references and index.
        ISBN 978-1-57731-095-2
        1. Aromatherapy for children. I. Title.

     RJ53.A76 W67 1999
     615'.321'083—dc21   98-032427

ISBN 978-1-57731-095-2
First New World Library printing, March 2000
Printed in the USA on acid-free paper

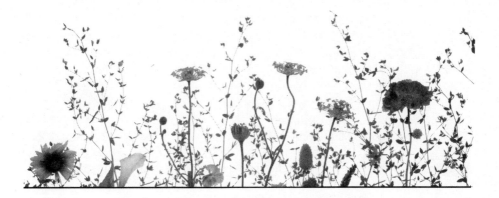

❧

Special thanks go to all the parents who have trusted my judgments and advice, brought their children to my practice, used my books for healing, and passed on the information to friends and family, at school gates and playgrounds. Many I have never met, but they have kindly written to me over the years, telling me their personal stories and passing on valuable comments.

❧

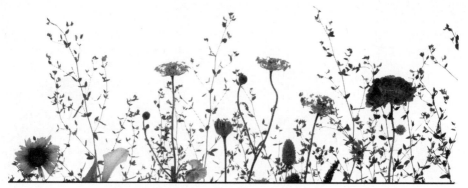

Table of Contents

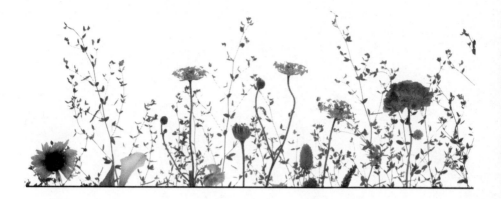

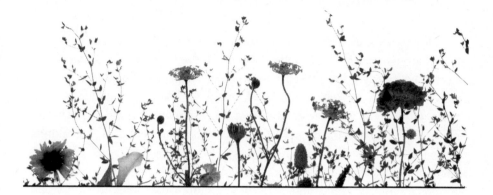

Foreword

Nothing in the world is more precious to us than our children, and it's a daunting responsibility to care for them. We all rely heavily on the medical professions to keep our children healthy, and we should continue to take advantage of all the benefits modern medicine can offer us. But there are times when help is not available, when we have to fall back on our own resources, and take the care of our children into our own hands.

Many of us may simply prefer to use natural medicines whenever we can. There is certainly a trend towards natural medicine, not only among the general public, but within the medical professions. The advantages of integrative medicine are increasingly appreciated, as natural remedies are used alongside conventional medical treatment.

There's nothing new in natural medicine. From earliest times parents around the world have taken from nature the herbs and plants they needed to care for the health of their children. Aromatherapy is a modern version of that long tradition of using what's available, natural, and works. These days we have scientific papers to back up empirical evidence, and instead of long treks into the countryside to collect healing plants, we have convenient dropper bottles full of plants' healing essential oils. Aromatherapy offers great convenience and flexibility, and there's never been a better time to take advantage of nature's fragrant pharmacy.

In my practice as a clinical aromatherapist I've seen the wonderful healing effect of aromatherapy and essential oils on children. Friends and family have used my knowledge, and passed it on to their friends and family. I constantly hear of the positive results this has brought to adults and children alike. Readers all over the world who have used the information in my books kindly write and tell me how much aromatherapy has helped them or their children. I'm also a consultant to the aromatherapists working with The Children's Society in England, to relieve the difficulties faced by children who are physically or emotionally disadvantaged. These children have hills to climb, and aromatherapy helps them. Yet I did not plan to write a book for children. My editor, Becky Benenate suggested it, and I had to think long and hard.

There has been talk that aromatherapy should only be used by people trained in the profession. Part of this argument maintains that general readers aren't capable of following instructions, and shouldn't be encouraged to get involved in something they know nothing about.

As I wondered about all this, the phone rang. It was my brother. The previous evening he'd gone to a dinner party where another guest, a woman, said aromatherapy saved her child's life. Her baby was born prematurely with severe health difficulties. The doctor at the hospital said there was nothing further they could do, take your baby home and prepare for the worst. The mother was devastated. Then a nurse came and showed her a copy of an aromatherapy book and said "go and buy a copy and follow the instructions." She did this, and the baby is now a healthy two year old. "What was the book?" someone asked, and she replied *The Complete Book of Aromatherapy & Essential Oils* — one of my earlier books. When my brother told the lady that I am his sister, she asked him to tell me "thanks." That's why he'd called.

It was a message to me. Aromatherapy can be beneficial to children's health, and if people are informed, they can use it to help their children. So, I offer you here my knowledge, however there's another side to this — you, the caregiver. You're the person who is going to carry out the instructions, and I rely on you to follow them correctly. Also, please take care to find a reputable supplier of essential oils. If you do these things, I have confidence you too will discover the healing power of essential oils.

When I was a little girl my mother treated everyday ailments with herbs and healing plants, administered around the kitchen table. To older generations in Europe this was normal. Not everyone could afford to go to the doctor every time something was wrong with a child. For them, it was not a question of natural medicine being an alternative. Indeed, at one time, modern medicine was the alternative.

The tradition of natural medicine lives on in modern aromatherapy. Those of us who have been using essential oils for a long time, and have seen our children grow up and have children of their own, take great pleasure in the fact that younger generations now use essential oils, and recommend them to their friends. One drop of essential oil, performing some task of healing, falls into the pool of general knowledge, and ripples out, touching others. This is how aromatherapy is today. The ripples are getting stronger, and spreading further, because aromatherapy works.

As a clinical aromatherapist, and working with others in the field, I know that individual children can benefit from aromatherapy — children of all ages, temperaments, and states of health. I finally came to the conclusion it would be wrong of me not to share knowledge which so many others have benefited from. Everything in aromatherapy is natural, a gift from God. The essential goodness of essential oils cannot be denied. They are powerful, that is true, and we must always regard them with respect. If we do that, they will help us through some of the hardest times we shall have to face, when our precious children are not well.

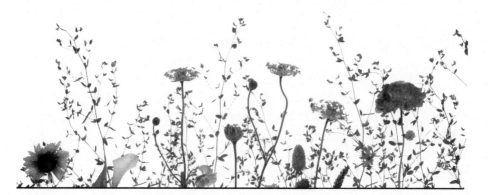

Introduction

What's So Great about Aromatherapy?

Every parent has been in the position of having a sick child to care for with no available help. It's a horrible feeling. Perhaps the doctor is not available until the following morning, or you are snowed in and can't go and get help. With aromatherapy, however, you're not helpless; there's something you can do — something that's been shown to work through long term use, and through a great deal of scientific research. As well as helping out in emergencies, aromatherapy lets you think proactively about the long term health of your child.

The essential oils used in aromatherapy are 100 percent pure, natural essences distilled from a variety of plants. These are very concentrated substances, measured in drops. Using just one drop is not unusual. The essential oils come from flowers, leaves, roots, resin, seeds, fruits, and wood, depending on the plant species.

The first essential oil people often buy is lavender because it's so versatile. It can help with the healing process of cuts and grazes, and is the best thing for burns. Plus it smells nice and can be diffused around the home, or put in the bath for when you want to relax and have a good sleep. That's just one oil. Add a few more and you get not only their individual properties, but the fact that when two or more essential oils are mixed together, they make a new therapeutic composition, able to perform tasks not possible for the individual oils on their own. So you get two things — individual oils, and a whole array of mixes. Combining essential oils into unique blends gives aromatherapy depth, richness, and tremendous flexibility.

You will discover that the healing power of nature, in the form of aroma-therapy, is very easy to use at home. Because the essential oils come in volatile liquid form, there are lots of ways they can be used. The only things you will need in addition to essential oils are a few small empty bottles, some carrier oil like almond oil, and a diffuser. Most other things you might need are likely to be in your home already.

In terms of therapeutic potency, most essential oils have a shelf-life of approximately two years. However, the therapeutic properties of the citrus oils, such as lemon, are said to diminish after six months. But even when an essential oil has lost its therapeutic vibrancy, it can still be used in all sorts of ways. Lemon, for example, can be used in a room diffuser or air-freshening spray, or even to wipe down kitchen surfaces, or freshen the laundry.

There's no telling when a child might get sick. They can walk out of their bed in the middle of the night and complain of an ache or wake up with a cough. With aromatherapy, it's often possible to deal with the situation right then and there. That's a great relief when you have a crying child asking for your help. Essential oils are not a cure-all and won't be able to assist with every crisis you'll have to deal with as a parent, but they can deal with more than you think they can. As you discover this, you'll wonder how you ever managed without them.

Aromatherapy for the
Healthy Child

Part 1

The Essentials of Nature's Healing Tools

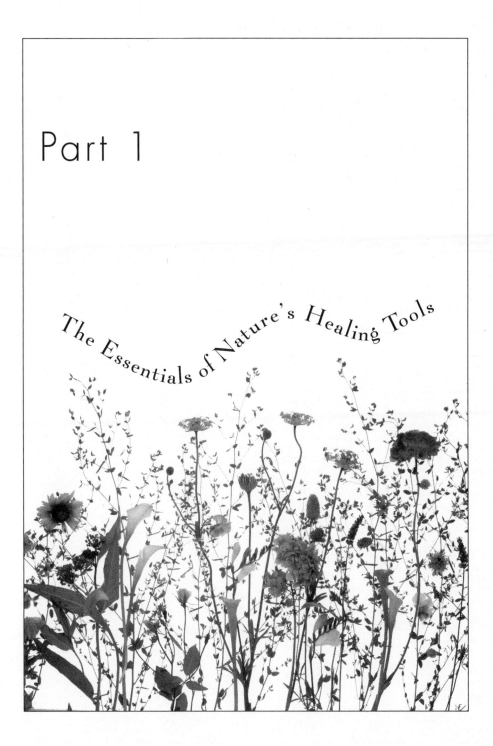

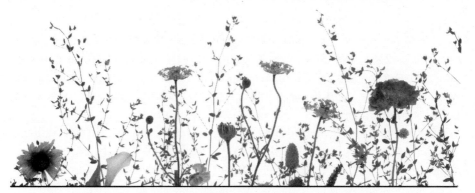

CHAPTER ONE **The Essentials**

"The Essentials" offers you some of the principles to using home-help aromatherapy for children successfully and safely. In chapter 4, "The A–Z of Conditions," there are particular instructions to follow when using essential oils specific to a condition. When using aromatherapy for children more generally, however, there are basic directions and important facts you need to know. This information is outlined below.

Essential oils are pure plant essences. They are distilled from flowers, leaves, seeds, fruit, roots, resin and wood. See Essential Oils — Nature's Healing Tools.

Only some essential oils are suitable for children. See pages 5–8 for a chart showing which oils you can use as a child increases in age.

Essential oils used correctly do not conflict with medically prescribed drugs. They can be used alongside other treatments. Integrative medicine is the way of the future.

Essential oils are used externally — on the outside of the body. Use them in body oils, lotions, creams, gels, baths, showers, foot baths, compresses, dressings, and in the sponging down method. You can diffuse them in the atmosphere, spray them in the air, and inhale them from a tissue. See pages 15–22 for how to use the different methods.

Essential oils are diluted in different strengths. Depending on what condition your child has, and their age, you might need to dilute just one single drop in 1 ounce of vegetable oil, 1 tablespoon, 1 dessertspoon, 1 teaspoon, $\frac{1}{2}$ teaspoon, $\frac{1}{4}$ teaspoon, or 1 drop of vegetable oil. There is a huge variation in the degree of dilution, depending on the effect that's required.

Blend two or more essential oils together before diluting. When using two or more essential oils, mix them all together in the empty bottle so they can amalgamate, then add the diluting carrier oil. When using a single oil, it doesn't matter if you put them in the bottle first, then add the carrier oil, or put the carrier oil in the bottle first, and add the essential oil after.

Sometimes just one or two drops of a complex mix of essential oils are used. Blends of many oils are often more potent than single oils. In those blends, some essential oils might contribute 1 or 2 drops, while others are needed in larger amounts, say 5 or 6 drops. A mix is thus made up of both different essential oils, and different amounts of essential oil. When the mix is complete, we can take from it how much we need. It could be just one drop, but it will be a complex drop, combining many properties.

We often prepare more diluted oil than we intend to use. For example, in the case of baby's colic, only 1 drop of colic mix is needed in $1/2$ a teaspoon of vegetable oil. Of this, only a very small amount will be used. The rest will go to waste. However, there's no other way to do it. You can't measure less than one drop of essential oil, so to get the right proportions of essential oil-to-vegetable oil, we have to make more than we need.

Essential oils and diluted blends are delicate. Keep all pure essential oils and all diluted oils in a cool, dry, dark place — away from sunlight.

Essential Oils — Nature's Healing Tools

Essential oils are distilled from certain healing plants, usually by steam distillation. Depending on the plant, the essential oil is produced in the petals, roots, leaves, seeds, fruit rind, bark, wood, or resin. Essential oils are produced all around the world for use in medicines, foods, drinks, perfumery and, of course, aromatherapy.

Almost all essential oils are antiseptic, and individual oils have their own particular healing characteristics. Some have strong antibacterial properties, others are antiviral, antifungal, antiinflammatory, or antispasmodic. Some are calming, others are stimulating. Each essential oil has a healing profile, comprised of several characteristics, that is unique to itself.

When using essential oils on children, it's important to recognize that some essential oils are not suitable for them. This might be because the essential oil has hormonal properties, or it may be too powerful for the weaker constitution of children. If using an essential oil for a particular condition, only use the oils recommended in that section of "The A–Z of Conditions." For more general purposes, use the essential oils recommended for your child's age-group, which can be found in the following chart.

What's in a Name?

The name of essential oils is very important. There are many different types of eucalyptus or camomile, for example, each with its own particular healing properties. When I recommend "camomile roman," don't confuse it with "camomile german," or ormenis flower, which some people call "camomile maroc." Please take care to use the correct essential oil for the job. This is particularly important in the case of children. "Thyme" oil is not generally recommended for children because it is so strong, but there's an alternative in the related "thyme linalol," which is excellent for use on children.

Essential Oils for General Purposes			
Child's Age	Essential Oils	Basic Carrier Oils	Small Additions — Base Oils
Newborn	camomile roman, camomile german, lavender, mandarin, dill	almond (sweet)	jojoba, wheatgerm
2–6 months	camomile roman, camomile german, lavender, mandarin, dill, eucalyptus radiata, neroli, tea tree, geranium, rose otto	almond (sweet)	jojoba, wheatgerm
7 months–1 year	camomile roman, camomile german, lavender, mandarin, dill eucalyptus radiata, neroli, tea tree, geranium, rose otto, palmarosa, petitgrain, niaouli, tangerine, cardamom	almond (sweet)	jojoba, wheatgerm, calendula (infusion)

Essential Oils for General Purposes

7 months–1 year	camomile roman, camomile german, lavender, mandarin, dill, eucalyptus radiata, neroli, tea tree, geranium, rose otto, palmarosa, petitgrain, niaouli, tangerine, cardamom	almond (sweet)	jojoba, wheatgerm, calendula (infusion)
2–5 years	camomile roman, camomile german, lavender, mandarin, dill eucalyptus radiata, neroli, tea tree, geranium, rose otto, palmarosa, petitgrain, niaouli, tangerine, cardamom, thyme linalol, ginger, lemon, grapefruit, ravensara, ormenis flower, coriander, helichrysum, yarrow	almond (sweet)	jojoba, wheatgerm, calendula (infusion), red carrot
6–8 years	camomile roman, camomile german, lavender, mandarin, dill eucalyptus radiata, neroli, tea tree, geranium, rose otto, palmarosa, petitgrain, niaouli, tangerine, cardamom, thyme linalol, ginger, lemon, grapefruit, ravensara, ormenis flower, coriander, helichrysum, yarrow, bergamot, marjoram, eucalyptus, citriodora, myrtle, pine, ho-wood, myrrh, spikenard, orange	almond (sweet), apricot, peach kernel, camellia, sunflower, grapeseed	jojoba, wheatgerm, calendula (infusion), red carrot

Essential Oils for General Purposes			
9–11 years	camomile roman, camomile german, lavender, mandarin, dill, eucalyptus radiata, neroli, tea tree, geranium, rose otto, palmarosa, petitgrain, niaouli, tangerine, cardamom, thyme linalol, ginger, lemon, grapefruit, ravensara, ormenis flower, coriander, helichrysum, yarrow, bergamot, marjoram, eucalyptus, citriodora, myrtle, pine, ho-wood, myrrh, spikenard, orange, frankincense, cypress, melissa, elemi, ylang ylang	almond (sweet), apricot, peach kernel, camellia, sunflower, grapeseed	jojoba, wheatgerm, calendula (infusion), red carrot
9–11 years	camomile roman, camomile german, lavender, mandarin, dill eucalyptus radiata, neroli, tea tree, geranium, rose otto, palmarosa, petitgrain, niaouli, tangerine, cardamom, thyme linalol, ginger, lemon, grapefruit, ravensara, ormenis flower, coriander, helichrysum, yarrow, bergamot, marjoram, eucalyptus, citriodora, myrtle, pine, ho-wood, myrrh, spikenard, orange, frankincense, cypress, melissa, elemi, ylang ylang	almond (sweet), apricot, peach kernel, camellia, sunflower, grapeseed	jojoba, wheatgerm, calendula (infusion), red carrot

Room Method Oils		
With children, the following essential oils can only be used in the room methods, such as diffusers and sprays. Unless otherwise indicated in this book, only use with children over 3 years of age.		
oregano cinnamon	thyme red citronella bay	clove fennel

Buying and Storing

If you are planning to use essential oils with children, it is crucial to find a good supplier of pure, organic if possible, essential oils. Many essential oils sold today are not what they seem. They could be chemical copies made to mimic the aroma of a particular essential oil. Or, they could be industrial quality essential oils that are too old to have any therapeutic qualities left. They might be pure oils, but already diluted in a vegetable oil — and not suitable for the purposes outlined in this book. Some are sold as "fragrant oils" or even "aromatherapy oils," and are intended for use as sweet-smelling body oils or room fragrances. These sweet-smelling oils are totally different from the healing tools of essential oils.

Due to the growth of aromatherapy in recent years, there are now many good suppliers of pure essential oil who can supply you with the essential oil you need, and often by mail order. Most health stores will sell 100 percent pure essential oil, and if you have any difficulty, look at small ads in health magazines where mail-order suppliers are likely to be found.

Essential oils should be supplied and kept in dark glass bottles that have a dropper-stopper. Always read the label carefully, checking that it says "100 percent pure essential oil." Ideally, the Latin name should be printed on the label, along with a "sell-by" date — which might be two years hence. Don't buy essential oils that are displayed on shelves that catch the sun. Essential oils need to be stored in a cool, dark place, and if the management of a store aren't aware of that elementary rule, they're unlikely to have taken the trouble to source a quality supplier.

Keep your essential oils and blends somewhere dark and cool, out of a humid atmosphere. Bathrooms are often full of damp steam and are not a good place to keep them. You have to think about the children too, and put the essential oils somewhere where they can't be reached. Wooden storage boxes especially made for essential oils are available and are the most convenient way to store them. Put the box, or other container, on a high shelf out of reach of inquisitive little minds and hands.

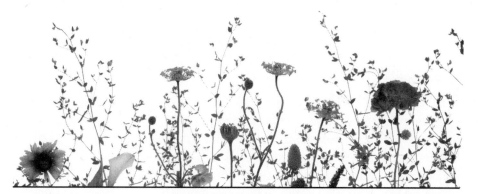

CHAPTER TWO **Using Essential Oils**

Hydrolats, Essential Oil Waters, and Infused Oils

Throughout this book I refer to "hydrolats," essential oil "waters," and "infused" oils. They are all products which include some elements of the healing properties of the essential oils found in plants. Hydrolats can't be made at home, but can be purchased from specialist suppliers. Essential oil waters are made with essential oils and they can be used, in some cases, in place of hydrolats.

Hydrolats

A great deal of water is used in the process of essential oil distillation, and it's often sold as a by-product of the manufacturing process — a hydrolat. Rose water and orange-flower water, which are used in beauty preparations and cooking, are diluted hydrolats. Herbal medicine uses these and other hydrolats, such as lavender, tea tree, and camomile.

It's only the water-soluble components in plants that become imbued in the water used in the distillation process. Consequently, hydrolats should not be thought of as watered down essential oils, because they don't contain all the components that essential oils do. Hydolats very often smell quite different from the plant or the essential oil.

Hydrolats have antiseptic properties, and have their own unique uses. They can be used to spray rooms, put on bed clothing, as well as on compresses. They often have a delicious fragrance. Hydrolats have to be bought like an essential oil. If your supplier doesn't sell them you may be able to get them through an herbalist.

Essential Oil Waters

The water-infusion method creates an essential oil water, which could be used if a hydrolat is unavailable. Pour $1/_2$ pint of boiling water into a heat-proof bowl. Then add 6–10 drops of your chosen essential oil. Cover the bowl completely, so the cooled, condensed water falls back into the bowl. Then pour the mixture through an unbleached, paper coffee filter, to take out the globules of essential oil. Leave it to cool, then bottle.

Infused Oils

Infused oils can be made at home and there are two ways to make them. The first way is to use a jelly jar or other container that can be kept tightly sealed, and fill it with whatever plant material you want to use, such as lavender, camomile, marigold, or calendula. Use the part of the plant that contains the essential oils. (For complete details on essential oils profiles see *Essential Aromatherapy: A Pocket Guide to Essential Oils & Aromatherapy* by Susan Worwood.) Pack in as much as you can, then fill the jar with a good, organic vegetable oil, such as sunflower, grapeseed, or almond oil. Put the lid on tightly, and put the jar somewhere in the sun, like a window sill. Shake the bottle every day. After at least 48 hours, strain the oil again. To really get all the bits out, strain the oil through an unbleached paper coffee filter. It's thick, so this will take some time. To make the oil stronger, use the same oil and add more fresh plant material, and repeat the process. Carry on until you get the aroma as strong as you want it.

The second method involves putting the flower heads or other plant material in a jar with the oil, as above and, after sealing the jar, gently heating the oil and the plant together. This is done by putting the jar into a few inches of water in a pot, on the stove. Use low heat — there should be no bubbling or boiling. Strain as usual.

Other Ingredients

Other ingredients and equipment used will be discussed throughout this book; below is further information about them:

Alcohol: Use only pure, organic, food-quality alcohol, or vodka.

Aloe Vera: The aloe vera plant has renowned healing properties. It has long, hard, thick, spiky leaves. In the center of each leaf is a sticky gel-like substance, that can be taken out as required. The plant grows easily on sunny window ledges, requires little maintenance, and propagates itself — producing more baby plants which can be repotted. The plant provides an easily accessible, fresh source of aloe vera, which is the best form to use. However, aloe vera can also be purchased in water or gel form. Aloe vera is an antiinflammatory, and can soothe the skin and help heal cuts, grazes, and burns, as well as ease insect bites.

Baking Soda: Sodium bicarbonate ($NaHCO_3$), known to most people as baking soda, is a sodium salt which softens water. It relieves itching and is soothing to the skin when used in the bath.

Bicarbonate of Soda: Sodium carbonate, also known as "washing soda" (Na_2CO_3).

Beeswax: Always use the pure, unbleached variety of beeswax. This is obtainable from health stores, specialist stores, beekeepers, and from some good quality drugstores and pharmacies.

Calamine Lotion: A pink or white pharmaceutical preparation for soothing and calming the skin. It can be found in drugstores and pharmacies.

Cider Vinegar: This must be organic if used to soothe and soften the skin. It can help restore the acid mantle of the skin and soothes irritation and stings.

Colloidal Silver: This is a specialized product, with strong antibacterial and antifungal properties. It is available from some health stores, and through certain network marketing companies.

Epsom Salts: This is used to help ease sore muscles and stiffness. It is not a water softener. It is available from most drug stores, pharmacies, and health stores.

Glucose Powder: A powdered form of glucose, found in most food outlets and drugstores.

Green Clay: This has long been used in European health and beauty preparations. The clay, taken directly from the ground, has healing properties. It is deodorizing, and can help in the healing of cuts and other skin problems.

Honey: Only use the very best you can find — a pure organic flower honey. Manuka honey is healing and highly recommended for the purposes outlined in this book.

Iodine: Easily found in drugstores and pharmacies.

Menthol Crystals: This is crystallized menthol, extracted from the mint plant family. It is available from drugstores and pharmacies.

Myrrh Tincture: Myrrh tincture is an alcoholic solution of myrrh. It's found in drugstores and pharmacies.

Oats/Oatmeal: Only use raw, organic oats or oatmeal, found in organic food stores and some supermarkets.

Rose Water: Produced in the distillation of rose oil. The most concentrated form is a hydrolat. When it is rediluted, it is called rose water. It's used in cooking and skin care for its skin softening and healing properties.

Salt: Salt is healing and cleansing. The salt referred to in this book is either sea salt or rock salt. The salt should contain as little chemical or additional substances as possible.

Vegetable-based Ointment: Usually available from health stores or organic food stores, but may be found in some drugstores.

Water: When water is mentioned as an ingredient — other than for baths and compresses — it means spring or distilled water.

Witch Hazel: Witch hazel is made from a bush, and comes in distilled, or infused form. It's a mild astringent with soothing and sting-relieving properties. It can be found in most drug stores, pharmacies, and supermarkets.

Zinc Oxide Cream: A cream that contains zinc, which is widely used as a skin healing medium. Easily available from drugstores and pharmacies.

Equipment Used

Bottles: Always keep essential oils and blends in dark bottles — either brown, green, or blue.

Hot Water Bottle: This refers to a large flat rubber bottle which you fill with warm water. It is preferable to use one with a cover made of soft material.

Muslin: Muslin is a very fine cheese cloth type of material. Try to find a pure cotton unbleached muslin, available from specialist material stores and some craft stores.

Paper Coffee Filters: This refers to the cone-shaped papers used to filter coffee. Use the unbleached paper variety.

Warm Bags: Warm bags contain wheat, corn, buckwheat, and other natural materials. This is covered in a material that can be heated in the microwave, or put in the refrigerator or freezer. They can be found in many department stores and health stores.

The Methods

There are two ways to use aromatherapy on children. You can use essential oils to get a child well — which is a home-help form of clinical aromatherapy and is the main subject of this book. And aromatherapy can be used simply to give a general sense of well-being — which is never far from our minds, and more elaborated upon in this chapter under Caring Touch Massage (see pages 30–32).

All essential oils should be sold with a dropper-hole insert already in place, which makes measuring easy. Essential oils differ in terms of their density and viscosity. The watery-type, like lavender, come out of the dropper-hole easily, while you have to be patient with the thicker type of essential oils, like sandalwood.

In chapter 4, "The A–Z of Conditions," there are recommended methods and instructions for the number of drops to use on children of different age groups. The amounts are very specific for a particular condition and are never a general rule. There are however, general guidelines for the amount of essential oil that should be used with a child of a particular age, for all the different methods, and they are given below.

Baths	Amounts to use*	
Run the bath as usual, then add the teaspoon of diluted essential oil, and swish the water around. Shut the door to keep the aroma in the bathroom. Use essential oils diluted in a small amount of vegetable oil, milk, or diluted milk powder.	Dilute in 2 teaspoons or 10 ml. of vegetable oil:	
	Newborn–6 months	1 drop, and use $^1/_4$ this amount
	6 months–2 years	1 drop, and use $^1/_2$ this amount
	2–5 years	1–2 drops, and use $^1/_2$ this amount
In baths, diluted essential oils are gentler on children's delicate skin.	6–10 years	1–3 drops
	11 and over	1–4 drops
	* Unless following instructions elsewhere in this book.	

Body Oil or Body Rub	*Amount to use**
Use the body oil or body rub like a body lotion — just smooth it on the skin. For suggested well-being blends, see Caring Touch Massage on page 31. If using one single essential oil, just add it to the base, vegetable, oil already in the bottle. If using two or more essential oils, put them into the empty bottle first, mix them well, by rolling the bottle between your hands, and then pour in the vegetable oil — up to the "shoulder" (not as far as the neck of the bottle), and roll again. See Blending on pages 23–27.	Dilute in 1 ounce of vegetable oil: Newborns 0–1 drop 2–6 months 1–2 drops 6–12 months 1–3 drops 1–4 years 1–5 drops 5–7 years 3–6 drops 8–12 years 5–9 drops 12 years and over 5–10 drops *Unless following instructions elsewhere in this book.

Clothing	*Amount to use**
Some essential oils will leave a mark on material, so only use this method if the clothes aren't valuable. It's a useful method to keep insects at bay. Put neat (undiluted) essential oil or diluted spray on socks, shoes, the bottoms of shorts, skirts, or trouser legs, or on the collar, sleeves, or cuffs of shirts and tops. This method is also useful for students who want to inhale a concentration-enhancing aroma when they're taking an exam — put it on the cuff of a long-sleeved shirt.	For children over 2 years only: 1 drop *Unless following instructions elsewhere in the book.

Compress	*Amount to use**
Put $^1/_2$ pint of water in a bowl, and add the essential oil (alternatively, use hydrolats or essential oil waters. Put the compress material in the water and leave it to soak for a short while. Then squeeze out the excess water, and place the compress over the area. Hold or tie it in place. Eye compresses should only be made with hydrolats or waters taking care that no substance gets into the eye. Always use 100 percent natural material for the compress, unbleached if possible, and large enough to cover the affected area when folded several times. Compresses can be used hot, warm, tepid, cool, or cold. Warmth increases the flow of blood to an area, cold restricts the flow of blood to an area.	For children over 2 years only: 2–4 drops *Unless following instructions elsewhere in the book.

Cotton Swab (Q-tip)	*Amount to use**
Put the undiluted essential oil (neat) onto a wet cotton bud, and apply directly to the affected area.	For children over 2 years only: 1 drop *Unless following instructions elsewhere in this book.

Diffusers/Burners	*Amount to use**
Diffusers/burners are two-tier objects, with a top bowl-like section for putting the water and essential oil, and a lower section for the tea-light candle which heats the water above. Put warm water in the upper bowl, light the candle below, then place your chosen essential oil/s onto the water.	*Up to 2 years* *1–2 drops* *2–5 years* *1–3 drops* *6–10 years* *1–4 drops* *11 and over* *1–5 drops*
As the candle heats the water, the essential oils and water evaporate. Keep an eye on diffusers to make sure the water does not evaporate before the candle goes out.	
If the water level is looking low, top it off with more warm water.	
Diffusers are usually made of ceramic or glass. If ceramic, make sure the water-bowl area is glazed — so you can wipe it with a cloth between use and clear away any gooey residue.	
There are also electrical diffusers/burners, with no candle section. Make sure you do not leave these plugged in after the water has evaporated.	
Nebulizers or oil vaporizers put a continuous fine spray of essential oil into the atmosphere. They were designed for clinical use and should not be used at home for children as the quantities of essential oil emitted and inhaled are far too high.	**Unless following instructions elsewhere in this book.*

Dressings	*Amount to use**
This method is used to help stop the spread of infection and to promote wound healing. The essential oil is put directly onto the dressing that is covering the affected area — such as Band-Aids (the inner, fabric part), or lint and gauze dressing. Leave the essential oil to dry before applying. This will prevent it stinging, but it will still be effective.	6 months and over only: 1–2 drops *Unless following instructions elsewhere in this book.

Face Oils	*Amount to use**
Face oils should only be used if there is a condition that requires it. Avoid the eye, mouth, and nose areas.	Dilute in $1/_2$ ounce of almond oil: 6 months–2 years 1 drop 3–5 years 1–3 drops 6–10 years 1–4 drops 11 and over 1–6 drops *Unless following instructions elsewhere in this book.

Foot Baths	*Amount to use**
Fill a large bowl with warm water and add 1 teaspoon of diluted essential oil, swishing it around before placing the feet in the bowl.	Dilute in 1 teaspoon of vegetable oil: 2–5 years 1 drop 6–10 1–2 drops 11 years and over 1–3 drops *Unless following instructions elsewhere in this book.

Humidifiers	*Amount to use**
Add the essential oil to the water in the humidifier. Essential oils can leave a sticky residue. This should not be a problem with the type of humidifier that hangs over radiators. However, the more complex electrical types should be assessed before use, to see whether any sticky essential oil residue might damage your machine.	Any age: 1–4 drops per pint of water *Unless following instructions elsewhere in this book.

Inhalation	*Amount to use**
Tissue or Handkerchief Method Put the essential oil onto a paper tissue or cotton handkerchief, and sniff from it when required.	2 years and over only: 1–2 drops *Unless following instructions elsewhere in this book.
Pillow Method This method is usually used to assist breathing or sleeping. Put the essential oil on a corner of the pillow, on the underside, away from the eyes. Some essential oils stain material, so use an old pillowcase. Alternatively, put the essential oil on a cotton ball and put it inside the pillowcase, away from the eyes.	6 months and over: 1–2 drops *Unless following instructions elsewhere in this book.
P.J.s Method (Pajamas) Before your child is ready for bed, put a drop of essential oil on the pajamas and allow it to dry. Put it at the back of the collar or on the inside of the chest.	6 months and over: 1 drop *Unless following instructions elsewhere in this book.

Lotions, Creams, and Gels	Amount to use*
Essential oils can be diluted in materials other than vegetable oils. Use nonperfumed lotion, cream, or gel, made of natural materials.	Dilute in 1 ounce of lotion:
Add the required number of essential oil drops suitable for the age of the child, and mix well.	Newborns 0–1 drops 2–6 months 0–1 drops 6–12 months 1–2 drops 1–4 years 1–5 drops 5–7 years 3–6 drops 8–12 years 5–9 drops 12 years and over 5–10 drops
	*Unless following instructions elsewhere in this book.

Room Sprays	Amount to use*
Put the warm water in a new plant-mister, and add the essential oil. Shake it vigorously, then spray high into the air. Avoid spraying over anything that could be damaged by the water droplets falling on it, such as wooden furniture or delicate materials.	3 months and over only: 10 drops to each $1/_2$ pint of lukewarm water
	*Unless following instructions elsewhere in this book.

Showers	Amount to use*
Only use the essential oils of camomile, lavender, or geranium with this method.	5 years and over only: 1–2 drops
Put the essential oil on a dry wash cloth, wet it thoroughly with water, then wipe the washcloth over the body while the shower is running.	
Avoid the face and genital areas.	*Unless following instructions elsewhere in this book.

Sponging Down	*Amount to use**
Put 2 pints of warm or lukewarm water in a bowl. Add the essential oil, and swish around well. Use the water to sponge down your child.	1–5 years 1–2 drops 6–10 years 1–3 drops 11 and over 2–4 drops *Unless following instructions elsewhere in this book.

Wash	*Amount to use**
Put the water in a bottle, add the essential oils, and shake well. Then pour though a paper coffee-filter and re-bottle. This prepared wash is useful for washing infected or other areas, such as cuts and grazes.	1 year and over only: 20 drops in a pint of warm water *Unless following instructions elsewhere in this book.

Water Bowl	*Amount to use**
Put a pint of boiling water into a heat-proof bowl and take it to the room where it is needed. Add the essential oil to the steaming water. Place the bowl in an area of the room where children and animals cannot reach it.	To a pint of water, add: Up to 2 years 1–2 drops 2–5 years 1–3 drops 6–10 years 1–4 drops 11 years and over 1–5 drops *Unless following instructions elsewhere in this book.

Blending

Blending is all about combining essential oils with a carrier oil, sometimes called a "base oil" or "vegetable oil." We blend essential oils and carrier oils together to dilute the essential oil, allowing it to be spread over a greater area of skin, at the low dosages required.

The list of carrier oils that follows contains only those used in this book. Some are used very often, while others are used only for particular conditions. Carrier oils have their own healing properties and any particular one might be more appropriate for certain conditions than others. By far the most useful carrier oil to have for use on children is almond, as it can be used in nearly all blending situations. Always try to buy the best quality carrier oils you can find — organic and cold-pressed.

Carrier Oils for Children		
Almond	Castor	Olive
Avocado	Evening primrose	Rosehip seed
Calendula (infused oil)	Grapeseed	Sesame seed
Camellia	Jojoba	St. John's Wort (infused oil)

How Much to Use?

How much essential oil and carrier oil you use partly depends on whether you're blending for a baby, infant, child, or adolescent. It also makes a difference whether you're blending for the Caring Touch Massage, when your child is well, or for a specific ailment when your child is ill. Each condition will require the essential oil to be diluted in different volumes of carrier oil and at different strengths. So, you could say there are no hard and fast rules, but there are general guidelines for health and healing home-use and these are:

Diluted in 1 Ounce (30 ml.) of Vegetable Oil:	
Age	**Essential Oil**
Newborn	1–2 drops
2–6 months	1–3 drops
6–12 months	1–4 drops
1–4 years	5–8 drops
6–7 years	5–10 drops
8–12 years	5–12 drops
12 years and over	10–15 drops

Under Essential Oil, you'll find two numbers — the minimum and the maximum. For chronic, long-standing, conditions always start with the minimum number of drops. If that doesn't seem to be helping, add an extra drop into the diluted oil, until you find the right dosage for your child. The higher numbers are the maximum recommended, and are for acute situations only.

There are no general guidelines to diluting when a child is ill, because there is no general illness! Each infection or disorder needs to be treated with essential oils specific to it, by an appropriate method, using a specific amount of essential oil and carrier oil. Across the many different types of conditions, there are huge variations in how much essential oil would be used. It also makes a difference how much you use depending on whether the condition has been going on for a long time and is "chronic," or has just happened and is "acute."

Chronic cases would use lower amounts of essential oil, working upward if required, depending on the severity of the condition. Besides all this, there are other factors to consider when deciding how much to use, such as the body weight of your child.

Body Weight: Throughout this book, suggested amounts of essential oil have been given for the average weight of a child at a certain age. However, as we all know, very few people are average. "Average" is where we meet, not where we are!

The more body fat a child has, the less essential oil can be absorbed into the body where it's needed. So, if your child is over 5 years of age and they're carrying a lot of extra body fat, or are very tall for their age, or have a heavy frame, move up to the amount recommendations of the next age group up.

Organ Maturity: One reason different amounts of essential oil are recommended for the different age groups is that their organs are at different stages of development. Compare the skin of a new born baby with that of a child who is 10 and you'll see a difference. The digestive system of a new born is only mature enough to take the nutrients out of mother's milk or specially formulated baby milk. As the child gets older, they can eat mashed-up food, but no big pieces they cannot yet digest. That will come later. And so it is, everything in it's time. Using essential oils on children requires more flexibility than when using them on adults, for the simple reason that children grow.

Acute or Chronic: Acute conditions are those which suddenly come on and require first aid. A chronic condition has been going on for some time. Throughout this book if you see a drops recommendation for a particular condition with two numbers, i.e., 3–5, use the lower number, 3 drops, on children with a chronic condition, and if that is not effective, add one more drop, see how that works, and so on, up to 5. If the condition is acute, the higher amount could be used right away, if appropriate.

Storing Blends: Put labels on all blends, saying who they were prepared for, the condition, the ingredients, and the date. This will eliminate any confusion in the future.

Diluted blends of essential oil should not be kept for a long time. The vegetable carrier oil will go rancid after a while. It's best to only make up the amount of diluted oil you will need to use for a week or two, and make up fresh oils as you need them.

Carrier Oils for Children

The following carrier oils have been suggested in different sections of this book. In general, almond oil is the best oil to use on babies and children of all ages, and when in doubt, use it. Some of the oils below might only have been mentioned once or twice in the book, because they are not everyday type of oils but good to use for specific conditions. Castor oil, for example, is helpful in cases of flaky skin, but you wouldn't use it for very much else.

Aside from vegetable oils, there are other mediums or carriers that essential oils can be diluted in. For a list of these, see The Methods page 15 earlier in this chapter.

Almond (Sweet Nut) Oil: This has emollient, softening, and nourishing effects on the skin and is very suitable for use with babies and children.

Avocado (Flesh) Oil: Used in combination with other carrier oils — use one-third of avocado combined with two-thirds of almond oil, unless otherwise directed in an instruction. Avocado can be found in refined form, or in its unrefined state — thick and deep green. It's very nourishing to the skin, and contains minerals and vitamins. It's used mainly for dry or flaky skin conditions.

Castor Oil: This is not often used in aromatherapy, but it is useful in small amounts for flaky skin and scalp conditions.

Camellia Seed Oil: This is used for its skin softening and nourishing effects. It can be used on its own or in combination with other carrier oils.

Evening Primrose: This is only used as an addition to other carrier oils and only in very small amounts. It helps repair damaged skin and keeps the skin healthy.

Grapeseed: This is used on its own, when a more astringent oil is required. It can be difficult to find organic grapeseed oil.

Jojoba Oil: This oil is considered to be more of a "liquid wax," and is very useful for certain conditions. It has a softening effect on the skin and is good for the scalp and hair. Only use small amounts in combination with other carrier oils.

Olive Oil: This is a good oil to use on dry skin and on skin that needs nourishing. It's a traditional healing oil, but the smell can overpower the aroma of the essential oils. Only use organically-grown, cold pressed, virgin olive oil.

Rose Hip Seed Oil: Use only very small amounts in combination with other carrier oils. This is a very regenerative healing oil, useful for scarring, and other skin conditions.

Sesame Oil: Sesame plays a big part in traditional healing systems, such as Indian Ayurvedic healing. It has a very strong odor that may overpower the essential oils.

Sunflower Seed Oil: The kind of sunflower oil sold as regular cooking oil is not suitable for the purposes of children's aromatherapy. But organic, cold pressed sunflower is easily available and can be used as a carrier oil for children. It has some emollient properties for the skin and contains essential fatty acids which can have a beneficial effect.

Infused Oils Used in This Book

Calendula Oil: Calendula oil is made from marigold flowers. It's an orange oil and the stronger the color, the better the oil. It has been used for centuries to heal the skin and is good for skin and scalp infections. It also has an application to help reduce scarring.

St. John's Wort: This is a red oil, produced in the same way as calendula oil. Although the flowers used are yellow, they turn the oil red. The stronger the color, the better the oil. It is useful for bruises, sprains, and swelling.

Safety First

These are the essential safety points to remember. Read through the whole list. You need to know all these things to be able to use essential oils safely.

Choosing Oils

- *There's no need to use essential oils on children unless a health condition requires it.* Although your child will certainly benefit from massage carried out for general well-being, don't use essential oils as a preventative, in the medical sense, unless in antiviral or antibacterial room sprays and diffusers or burners.
- *Essential oils for home care health purposes should be used for a maximum of ten days at a time.* A period of fourteen days should elapse between uses, unless otherwise instructed by a qualified practitioner.
- *Only use the essential oils that have been recommended for children.*
- *The essential oils recommended in this book should be used in the context in which they are indicated.* The range of essential oils in this book will cover almost everything that you will need to do.

The Sun and Essential Oils

- Certain essential oils should not be used before going in the sun, as they may make the skin more sensitive to the sun's ultraviolet rays. They are:

  Bergamot (*Citrus aurantium, ssp bergamia*)
  Grapefruit (*Citrus paradisii*)
  Lemon (*Citrus limonum*)
  Lime (*Citrus limette*)
  Mandarin (*Citrus reticulata*)
  Tangerine (*Citrus reticulata*)

Bottles

- Make sure the dropper stops are firmly in place.
- Make sure the tops are tightly screwed on.
- Write the purchase date on new bottles of essential oil so you will know how fresh they are.

Storage

- Store essential oils in glass bottles only.
- Store your essential oils and blends well out of the reach of children.
- Store essential oils and blends somewhere dark, in a dry atmosphere, away from any source of heat such as radiators.
- The citrus essential oils deteriorate more quickly than other types of essential oil, but will last longer by keeping them in the refrigerator.

Blends

- Before making blends, make sure all the equipment you use is sterile. You can do this by boiling the equipment or using baby sterile solution.
- Use thoroughly dry glass bottles for blends. If you leave even a tiny amount of water in a bottle after washing, or there is a lot of condensation in the air, the blend will deteriorate and turn cloudy.
- After making a blend, put a label on the bottle. It should have the name of the person the blend was prepared for, the complete list of ingredients, and the date it was prepared.

Skin

- Don't use essential oils neat (undiluted) on the skin, unless indicated to do so in the instructions for a particular condition.
- If your child has very sensitive skin, it's wise to do a skin test before using any new single oil or blend.
- If you accidentally splash neat essential oil onto your child wash the area well with soap and warm water.

Eyes

- Keep essential oils away from the eyes, neat or diluted, in any of the methods such as forehead compresses.

- If an essential oil gets into the eye, neat or diluted, wash the eye very thoroughly with water or an eye solution. Seek medical help if the eye still stings after being washed out.

By Mouth

- In aromatherapy essential oils are not generally taken orally, by mouth.
- If you find that your child has accidentally swallowed essential oil in any form, give them a large glass of milk to drink and visit an emergency room immediately.

Fire

- Essential oils are flammable and should be kept away from naked flames.

Solvents

- Some essential oils act as solvents, such as citrus oils. They can damage wood and delicate fabrics, and take the print off paper.

Epilepsy

- Talk to your child's physician if you have any concerns about using aromatherapy.
- Don't use stimulating oils such as:
  Rosemary (Rosmarinus officinalis)
  Hyssop (Hyssopus officinalis)
  Sweet fennel (Foeniculum vulgare)
  Sage (Salvia officinalis)
  Camphor (Cinnamomum camphora)
- Only use calming oils such as:
  Camomile roman (Anthemis nobilis)
  Lavender (Lavandula angustifolia)
  Jasmine (Jasminum officinale)
  Petitgrain (Citrus aurantium)
  Neroli (Citrus aurantium)
  Rose otto (Rosa damascena)
  Geranium (Pelargonium graveolens)

While Taking Medication

- If your child is taking medication, reduce the amount of essential oil used by half that recommended for their age group.

Caring Touch Massage

There's nothing better for any child than the loving, caring touch of a parent. It may be no more than a gentle touch or squeeze of the hand but it tells the child they are special. A simple stroke on the cheek lets a child know they are loved and cared for. When they fall over we reach out and rub their knee better, or cuddle them in our arms. These are the everyday forms of touch we instinctually use with our children — and they thrive on it.

Research has shown that massage can help children's growth, both physically and emotionally. In hospitals, premature babies show that touch, even the touch of a single finger, can make a difference in their health. It is evident — children need a caring touch.

There can be no better way to promote health in your child than to give them regular massages, and you don't need to take a two-year course to learn how to do it. You don't need to use any deep-tissue massage techniques, just use very gentle stroking movements. Even with a light touch massage, always move your hands around your child's body, in the direction toward the heart, because it's the way the blood flows. All this means in practical terms is that your hands need to work from wrist to shoulder, and ankle to thigh. On the body, again work toward the heart. Good areas to massage are the back, upper abdomen, legs, feet, arms, and hands.

Essential oils are a bonus when it comes to massage. They provide great fragrances, they're natural and healthy, and can uplift the spirit. To make a massage oil, all you need is a clean, empty one ounce bottle, the carrier oil, and your essential oils. Use the following amount of essential oil, depending on the age of your child, in one ounce of vegetable carrier oil — almond is best.

Dilute in 1 Ounce (30 ml.) of Vegetable Oil:	
Age	*Essential Oil*
Newborns	0–1 drop
2–6 months	0–1 drops
6–12 months	1–2 drops
1–4 years	1–5 drops
5–7 years	3–6 drops
8–12 years	5–10 drops

You could use a single oil of your choice or a blend. When using a single oil all you have to do is put the essential oil drop or drops into the bottle of almond oil. When making blends, you have to mix the essential oils together first, to get the blend right. From this mix you take the appropriate number of essential oil drops you need and put them in the almond or other carrier oil. I find the best way to blend the essential oil and carrier together, is to roll the bottle between the palms of your hands. Here are a few blends that will give pleasure to both you and your child.

Caring Touch Massage Blends

Mix the essential oils together. Use the correct number of drops for your child's age group, diluted in almond oil.	
SLEEPY TIME	4 drops lavender 2 drops camomile roman
REFRESHING	3 drops lemon 2 drops petitgrain
ANGELIC	3 drops rose otto 2 drops neroli
FLOWERY	4 drops mandarin 2 drops geranium
CALMING	2 drops petitgrain 3 drops neroli

The Caring Touch Massage has an additional bonus — aromatic bonding. The aroma you choose to use during the massage of your child will be associated in your child's mind with times spent being relaxed and having a special time with their parent. The more regular your massages, the stronger the association will be. If your child smells the same aroma in another context, away from the place of massage, they will be reminded of the massage and the emotions that went with it — comfort, reassurance, and relaxation. This is an aromatic bond between you and your child, something that reminds your child of you, and you of your child.

This aromatic bonding can also be used to comfort small children, especially one separated from their parents, on the first day of starting kindergarten, for example. There are many times when small children have to be separated from their parents unwillingly and they can feel insecure and even afraid. To help ease the discomfort of separation, the aromatic link between parent and child can be used. Take a little smear of the same essential oil you use in your caring touch massage oil, and dab it on a tissue or cotton handkerchief, for your child to smell during the day. If your child is very young, the caretaker could just hold the tissue briefly under your child's nose. The aroma should remind your child of you and give some comfort and reassurance. The message of the massage lives on.

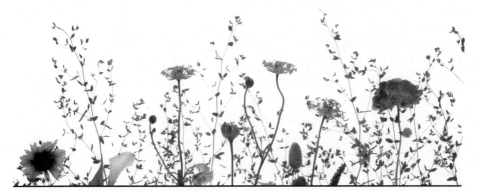

CHAPTER THREE **The Basic Care Kit for Children**

"The Basic Care Kit for Children" contains information about the twelve most useful essential oils to have in the home. With these oils in your first aid cabinet most conditions can be dealt with effectively. There are other oils of course, that are very useful, particularly for certain conditions. These are what you might call the extras, the ones I would want in the home, if I already had the twelve core basic kit oils. A basic care kit also needs some carrier oil and a few small, clean, empty bottles. Most of the equipment you may need is probably in your home already, such as cotton wool, Band-Aids, dressings, and a bowl. The only extra thing you may need is a diffuser.

With the basic tools of aromatherapy, you can take your children's basic care kit even further, and make things for the first aid cabinet. At the end of this section you'll find the recipes for making your own: Antiinfectious Air Spray; First Aid Washing Mix; Antiseptic Skin Spray; Antiseptic Antifungal Powder; Herbal Healing Infused Oils; Natural Salves and Ointments; Antiseptic Ointment; Chest Congestion Ointment; Baby Oil; and Baby Powder.

First, let us look at our children's basic care kit — the twelve most useful essential oils to have in the home for children, with the ailments the oils can help toward healing, either singly, or when in combination with others. It may be that the essential oil helps, not with the condition itself, but with one or more of the symptoms. For more information, please refer to the specific condition in chapter 4, "The A–Z of Conditions."

These essential oils are not listed in any particular order. Which oils you'll find most useful will depend on the age of your child, and the condition they have now or the ailments they are prone to.

Basic Care Kit — Essential Oils

◔ **Lavender** (*Lavandula angustifolia*)
(antiinfectious; antibacterial; antiinflammatory)
cuts, grazes, burns, promotes wound healing, psoriasis, eczema, sunburn, insect bites, headache, migraine, insomnia, rashes, nervous conditions, anxiety, tension

◔ **Tea Tree** (*Melaleuca alternifolia*)
(antiinfectious; antibacterial; antimicrobial; antifungal; antiinflammatory)
rashes, insect bites, nail fungus, ringworm, thrush, head lice, sore throats, boils, bronchial congestion, scabies, ulcers, wounds, cold sores, thrush, acne, bronchitis

◔ **Camomile Roman** (*Anthemis nobilis*)
(antibacterial; antiinflammatory; antispasmodic)
pain relief, fevers, skin problems, rashes, eczema, teething pain, muscular spasm, calming, helps nervousness, pain relief, insomnia, constipation

◔ **Camomile German** (*Matricaria recutita*)
(antiinflammatory; antispasmodic; antibacterial)
skin problems, asthma, eczema, arthritis, acne, ulceration's, fever, wound healing, nervousness, digestive complaints

◔ **Thyme Linalol** (*Thymus vulgaris, type linalol*)
(antibacterial; antiviral; antiinfectious; antifungal)
all infections; including viral, mucus congestion, colds, flu, muscular pain, arthritis, bronchitis, pneumonia, tuberculosis, thrush, coughs, throat infections, warts, pain relief

◔ **Ravensara** (*Ravensara aromatica*)
(antiviral; antibacterial; antiinfectious)
colds, flu, bronchitis, diarrhoea, fever, cold sores, sinusitis, whooping cough, herpes, chickenpox, measles, muscular pain, swollen lymph glands

✑ **Niaouli** *(Melaleuca quinquenervia)*
(antibacterial, antiparasitic, antiinfectious, antiviral)
colds, coughs, bronchitis, sinusitis

✑ **Cardamom** *(Elettaria cardamomum)*
(antispasmodic)
indigestion, flatulence, muscular cramps, fatigue, muscular spasms, catarrh, sinus headaches, constipation

✑ **Mandarin** *(Citrus reticulata)*
(antispasmodic)
convalescence, digestive problems, nervous tension, irritability, constipation, insomnia, anxiety

✑ **Eucalyptus Radiata** *(Eucalyptus radiata)*
(antiinfectious, antibacterial, antiinflammatory)
bronchitis, catarrh, coughs, colds, flu, fever, sinusitis, headaches, asthma, insect bites, rashes, acne

✑ **Helichrysum** *(Helichrysum angustifolium)*
(analgesic; antibacterial)
bronchitis, analgesic, pain relief, bruising, coughs, arthritis, circulation problems

✑ **Petitgrain** *(Citrus aurantium)*
(antispasmodic)
spots, boils, nervousness, insomnia, anxiety, stress, calming

Extra Basic Care Kit Essential Oils

Aside from the twelve listed above, there are other essential oils that are also very useful to have in your children's basic care kit. I've listed them in order of preference. By this I mean if I had to choose the most useful, the one at the top of the list would come first. The second oil on the list, reading downwards, would be the second most useful, and so on.

Geranium *(Pelargonium graveolens)*   **Rosemary** *(Rosmarinus officinalis)*
Palmarosa *(Cymbopogon martinii)*   **Lemon** *(Citrus limonum)*
Manuka *(Leptospermum scoparium)*   **Bergamot** *(Citrus bergamia)*
Neroli *(Citrus aurantium)*   **Rose Otto** *(Rosa damascena)*

Things to Make for Your First Aid Cabinet

Antiseptic Skin Spray

For this spray you will need:

2 ounces of preboiled spring water
$1/_2$ ounce alcohol or vodka
5 drops lavender
10 drops tea tree
10 drops thyme linalol
5 drops camomile german

In a clean bottle combine the essential oils with the alcohol and shake as vigorously as you can. Then add half the water (1 ounce) a little at a time and continue shaking. Store for 48 hours. Then add the remaining water and leave for an additional 24 hours, shaking the bottle whenever you remember. Strain through an unbleached paper coffee filter and put in a sterile spray bottle.

First Aid Washing Mix

Put into a small dropper bottle:

30 drops lavender
30 drops tea tree
5 drops ravensara
5 drops eucalyptus radiata
20 drops bergamot

Use 2–6 drops of the mix in a small bowl of water to wash cuts and grazes. Do not apply neat to any open cut or graze.

Antiseptic Antifungal Powder

First combine the following. Use a blender or this could form into a lumpy mass.

$1/_2$ cup of green clay (a natural healing clay found in health food stores)
1 teaspoon of finely powdered thyme herb
1 teaspoon of finely powdered marjoram herb

When combined, slowly add:

15 drops tea tree
15 drops manuka
15 drops palmarosa

If the mixture is lumpy, just let it dry out completely, then crush it into a fine powder again.

Antiinfectious Air Spray

For this spray you will need:

4 ounces water
2 ounces alcohol (or vodka)
20 drops thyme linalol
5 drops cinnamon
5 drops clove
10 drops tea tree
10 drops lemon

Put the essential oils into the alcohol, then add the oil/alcohol mixture to the water and leave it to stand for 24 hours. Transfer to a new plant mister, and spray into the air. Avoid letting the droplets fall on any polished wooden surfaces, delicate materials, or other materials that could be damaged by the water or other ingredients.

Herbal Healing Infused Oils

If you want to try making some of your own preparations instead of purchasing them, different herbs growing in your garden can be used to make healing herbal infused oils. These can't be used as a substitute for essential oils in any of the condition methods in this book, because the strength and properties are different, but infused oils can be used on their own, or as a substitute for vegetable carrier oils. Some of the most useful herbal infusions are:

Calendula	St. John's Wort
Melissa	Comfrey
Rosemary	Marjoram
Lavender	Rose
Camomile	

Lavender, rose, and camomile can be usefully included in massage oils for very young children. They can also be used as skin care preparations.

When making infusions, only use fresh, organically grown flowers or herbal materials and organically produced, cold-pressed vegetable oils. The oil you use is important, as this is what will be applied to your child's skin. Almond oil, sunflower seed oil, olive oil, and sesame oil would be good choices for this method. Use almond for sensitive skins, and sunflower seed for older children.

Although olive and sesame oils have their own strong odors that are likely to mask the odor of the plant material, the plants' healing properties will remain intact.

Tear the plant material up; never use a metallic object as it can leech out some of the therapeutic properties of the plant. Put the herbs or plant material in a jar that has been sterilized by boiling water. Jelly jars with good screw caps, or bottles, can be used to store your oil. Then cover the plant material with your chosen organic oil such as almond.

Put the jar in a place that catches a lot of sun — a sunny window ledge is ideal. Shake the mixture as often as you can to help the healing properties of the herb transfer to the oil. Leave the jar in place for three to seven days. Then strain the oil, using a piece of fine muslin or an unbleached paper coffee filter. It can take a long time for the oil to seep through a paper filter but it is effective in catching all the plant residue. If you want an even more potent infused oil repeat the process using the same oil with fresh plant material.

Natural Ointments and Salves

You can make your own ointments and salves from scratch using beeswax and infused oil. To make a soft ointment you will need:

1 cup of infused oil (of your choice)
1/2 ounce of nonrefined beeswax
essential oils

First, put the beeswax into a bowl which is being gently warmed in a double boiler. (Put a small heat-proof bowl into water heating in a cooking pot.) When the beeswax is melted, pour in the oil, stirring all the time, to create a soft ointment. Finally, while still stirring, add your chosen essential oils, and blend them in well. Put the finished mix into jars, while still warm, put the lid on tightly, and leave to cool.

As an alternative method, purchase a vegetable-based, nonpetroleum, Vaseline type of ointment, and transfer a little to a small, clean, lidded, pot. To this, add some essential oil, and stir in well. Good oils would be antiseptic and antibacterial essential oils.

Antiseptic Ointment

Blend the following together well:

$^1/_2$ ounce of ointment
10 drops thyme linalol
5 drops ravensara
6 drops lavender

Chest Congestion Ointment

Blend the following together well:

$^1/_2$ ounce antiseptic ointment
10 drops ravensara
10 drops eucalyptus radiata
5 drops niaouli

Use a small amount each time, rubbed over the chest and back.

Baby Oil

Most baby oils are made from mineral-based products, which form a barrier preventing dampness reaching baby's skin. It is said that these oils cannot be absorbed by the skin. You may like to try this natural alternative based on jojoba oil, which is a natural wax:

$^1/_2$ ounce of jojoba oil
1 ounce of almond oil

Blend well together, then add:

1 drop geranium
1 drop petitgrain (or lavender)

Baby Powder

Baby powder can be made from simple ingredients that are a safe alternative to talcum powder that has been shown in some research to be potentially damaging to baby's health. You can choose which essential oil to use, from lavender, geranium, or petitgrain. Mix the following together in a blender:

1 ounce of arrow starch
1 ounce of corn starch

Then add into the blender:

2 drops of your chosen essential oil

Leave the mixture to dry, and use as you would a talcum powder.

The Cave Man Eating Plan

And finally, a very important ingredient that enhances any basic care kit for children is a healthy diet. Thousands of years ago there were no sugar-enhanced foods, no quickly prepared foods, no dairy foods, or wheat products. We don't know if children were healthier then, but we do know that adopting an eating plan based on the food that early humans ate is good for our children — especially those who have become unhealthy, and subject to pollution related disorders and oversensitivity to foods.

The Cave Man Eating Plan is very simple. If the food walks, swims, or flies, you can eat it. If it grows in the ground, or on a tree, you can eat it. If the food is organically grown, you can eat it; and if it's frozen, you can eat it. What you can't eat is precooked or packaged foods, candy, sodas, or artificially flavored foods.

Cutting these things from your child's diet is not as hard as it first seems. Meats and fish could be bought fresh or frozen and cooked with natural herbs or spices. Salt and pepper are allowed. Vegetables can be steamed, roasted, broiled, or eaten raw in salads of all types. Desserts can be made from frozen fruit juice — just put it in your blender and mix it with honey. Fruit can be eaten raw or baked in pies. Cook those cookies, but don't use prepared mixes, which may contain chemicals, and will certainly contain preservatives.

If dairy products are needed, get organic milk that contains nothing but milk. Eat organic butter, which is far better for children than chemically prepared spreads. Use cold-pressed organic oils for cooking. Make popsicles with pure fruit juice, and sodas with fruit juice and carbonated water.

Organic food may cost more, but you'll be saving by not buying all that junk food. Get the kids baking. Give them a basic recipe, and let their imaginations run wild.

After starting the Cave Man Eating Plan, it's been known for some children to have withdrawal symptoms as the chemical flavorings and preservatives are taken away. It's the same as someone giving up cigarettes, alcohol, or caffeine — the first few days are rough. Your child may be grumpy and irritable, particularly when they can't have their favorite soda. But do persevere with the Cave Man Eating Plan for at least six weeks, and then see if their breathing, skin, emotions, and behavior have improved. Does your child seem happier and less aggressive? Do they settle into homework more easily? Are there now more cuddles than arguments? After six weeks, you can give your child the occasional treat — a soda perhaps, a candy bar, or ice cream.

Ideally, the whole family should be following the Cave Man Eating Plan to show solidarity and support of the child it's intended for, and because they will benefit too. The rest is up to you. Until our children can make informed food choices at a later age, it is a parent's responsibility to see that, as "you are what you eat," children are fed well.

Part 2

Treating Children with Essential Oils & Aromatherapy

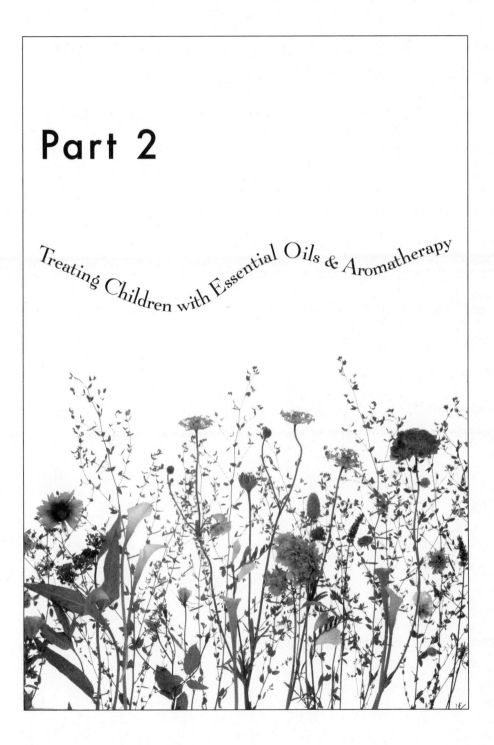

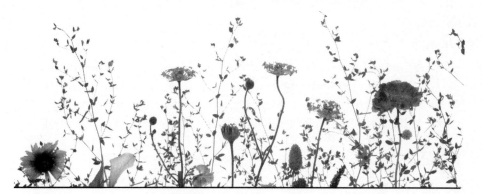

CHAPTER FOUR The A–Z of Conditions

This chapter outlines "The A–Z of Conditions" children experience with suggested essential oil methods of treatment. Some physical ailments are not conditions in themselves, so much as symptoms of a condition, such as cough, sore throat, fever, headache, rashes, vomiting, diarrhoea, and swollen lymph glands. If your child has one of these, especially if there are no other symptoms, look at that section to help find the possible cause.

That is not to say you should put yourself in place of a qualified medical practitioner. Medical help should be sought as needed. Get whatever help you can and think of essential oils and aromatherapy as nature's nursemaids, offering up their powerful goodness in the quest to keep our children well.

How to Use the A–Z Information

Symptoms

Under each entry several symptoms are listed. If your child has the condition, they might have just one of the symptoms on the list, several symptoms, or all the symptoms.

Symptoms will vary from child to child, depending on the severity of the condition, and on how the condition happens to manifest itself in your child — which will in part depend on your child's constitution, immunity, and home environment.

If your child has a symptom such as a cough, sore throat, fever, headache, rashes, vomiting, diarrhoea, or swollen lymph glands, read those sections also.

Methods

If you intend to carry out one of the methods, read all the instructions in the box. If using a particular method, refer to chapter 2, "Using Essential Oils," under the section titled The Methods, where further information may be found. If blending, also refer to chapter 2, under the section on Blending.

Essential Oils That Help

If you can't obtain the essential oils used in the methods outlined, refer to the Essential Oils That Help list. This contains some essential oils that can help the symptoms of the condition, not necessarily the condition itself.

Other Care

Often there is additional care that can be given to a child along with essential oil treatment. This may be something as simple as keeping the child warm or the suggestion of a breathing technique to help the child calm themselves.

When to Get Help

There will be times outlined in When to Get Help section, when it's important to get emergency medical care for the child. If ever in doubt, always seek professional medical help.

ACNE

There are two types of acne in children: newborn and adolescent.

Newborn Acne

Some babies are born with a facial rash that appears rather red and angry, with small red pimples covering their cheeks and nose. The rash occurs because certain hormones get passed from the mother while the baby is in the womb. It will disappear on its own within time, however, aromatherapy can help the process along. If possible get a diagnosis from the pediatrician before leaving the maternity unit.

There are three methods you can use, but in all cases first wash the baby's face by using a tiny pinch of very mild, pure soap, and rinse very thoroughly. To carry out the following methods by preparing hydrolats and teas please refer to page 11. In all cases, dab the area using a pure cotton ball.

Method One

This is the most effective method. Use lavender and camomile hydrolat.

Method Two

Using the Essential Oil Waters method: 1 drop each of lavender and camomile roman essential oils, in $\frac{1}{2}$ pint of water.

Method Three

Put 1 drop of lavender essential oil on an unused camomile tea bag, let it soak in, then allow to dry. When needed, put the tea bag in a cup, cover with boiling water, and put a saucer on top so no steam escapes. Allow to cool.

ADOLESCENT ACNE

According to the American Medical Association 85 percent of adolescents are affected with acne at some time. Acne is really heartbreaking for a teenager who wishes above all to look good to their peers. Acne can affect teenagers emotionally, leading to a loss of self-esteem and self-confidence. Also, anxiety and stress are increased, which can actually make the condition worse.

Adolescent or teenage acne is most often caused by increased hormonal activity. This creates an overproduction of sebum — the skin's natural oily moisturizer — where bacteria can flourish. Hair follicles, as well as pores, can become blocked by sebum. In most cases the acne clears up when the hormonal system harmonizes itself in early adulthood, but for many the problem goes on for years. Female adolescents have the added problem that their menstrual cycle can cause acne to erupt every month.

Signs and Symptoms

- can affect face, neck, back, and/or shoulders
- pimples, whiteheads, blackheads
- hair follicles that are infected appear reddened and can cause lumpy cysts to appear under skin, and these too can become infected

Over-the-counter acne preparations may increase the skin's sensitivity. They often leave a fine film on the skin that can attract more pollution and dirt to the area. Stronger formulations for the skin are generally prescribed and sometimes contain antibiotics. These may have side effects. Make sure your child is not using a friend's prescribed medication.

For some unlucky teenagers, acne can have lasting effects in the form of permanent scarring. Encourage your child to take care of their skin by cleaning it as gently as possible and keeping the skin exposed to fresh air. Cosmetics often cause more problems and may delay the healing process. Most important, there should be no squeezing or touching of the spots as this may lead to infection in areas, and can cause scarring and pitting in later life.

This is a disturbed and sensitive time for the skin, as it struggles to find a balance. Whatever the skin type, oily or dry, treat it as gently as possible. Wash with liquid soap, as pure and natural as you can find, rinse well, then apply one of the following tonics, and the moisturizer.

Skin Tonics	Moisturizer
Skin Tonic #1 *In equal proportions, mix together pure hydrolats of:* *Lavender* *Tea tree* *Rose* *Pour a small amount of the hydrolat onto cotton wool, and apply gently on the affected areas.*	*During the day try to leave the skin exposed to the air as much as possible. Use this moisturizer every evening. Mix the following:* *1 ounce of jojoba oil* *4 drops of rosemary* *4 drops of thyme linalol* *4 drops eucalyptus citriodora* *Apply a small amount on the face then dab off any excess by using a tissue.*
Skin Tonic #2 *Mix the following, and heat gently in a clean pot:* *4 ounces of rose water* *4 ounces of aloe vera juice* *5 drops of lavender* *4 drops of tea tree* *Leave to cool, then bottle. Apply a small amount onto a cotton swab and apply gently on the affected areas.*	

Blackheads	Other Spots
To remove blackheads, first steam the face. Don't squeeze them by hand but use a special blackhead extraction tool. Or have the job done professionally. After each one has been removed, dab with a little essential oil of lavender, applied with a cotton swab.	Dab some of the following on larger, pus-filled spots. First put the ingredients in a $^1/_2$ pint or larger bottle: $^1/_4$ bottle dry white wine 4 drops camphor 4 drops eucalyptus citriodora 2 drops lemongrass 2 drops thyme linalol 2 drops tea tree Shake well and use at least twice a day.

Essential Oils That Help

Lavender   Camphor
Rosemary   Eucalyptus citriodora
Tea tree   Bergamot
Thyme linalol

ARTHRITIS (JUVENILE RHEUMATOID)

Juvenile rheumatoid arthritis can affect children from as young as 2 years of age, right through to the teenage years. It's an auto-immune disease which means the body's immune or defense system attacks the body's own tissues instead of the usual enemy — invading micro-organisms and other such intruders. Depending on the type, rheumatoid arthritis causes inflammation of the joints or internal organs. There are three types:

a) Pauciarticular: less than four areas are affected, such as the knees, elbows, or ankles.

b) Polyarticular: when more than five areas or joints are affected, such as fingers, toes, hands, and feet.

c) Systematic: when both the joints and internal organs are affected.

The cause of juvenile rheumatoid arthritis is, as yet, not totally understood. Individual cases may vary and be caused by infection, genetic factors, or by damage to a joint.

Signs and Symptoms

- stiffness in the joints
- deformity of the joints caused by tightening of the tendons
- swelling, pain and, during later stages of an attack, some skin redness in the area
- symptoms can flare up and then go away

Aromatherapy should be seen as a complement to orthodox medical treatment — something in addition to it. The following methods may help ease the pain and stiffness. **Never massage joints or other inflamed parts of the body.** If using oils on painful areas, simply apply gently on the skin.

For Cold and Stiff Joints	*Inflammation Bath Blend*	*Compress Method*
The following mix can be applied to the joints every day. Also, it can be applied to joints before getting into a warm bath. Use only a small amount on painful areas. *First mix together:* *5 drops ginger* *5 drops marjoram* *5 drops myrtle* *2 drops clove* *4 drops helichrysum* *Then add to 2 ounces sesame oil and mix together.*	*Apply a small amount to each inflamed area, before getting in a warm bath.* *First mix together:* *10 drops camomile german* *5 drops camomile roman* *10 drops lavender* *10 drops eucalyptus citriodora* *Then add to 2 ounces almond oil and mix together.*	*Make up the blend as in Inflammation Bath Blend. Gently put a small amount on each affected joint. Then cover the area with a cold or warm compress — your child will tell you which is the most comfortable for them.*

Essential Oils That Help

Lavender

Camomile roman

Camomile german

Eucalyptus radiata

Eucalyptus citriodora

Geranium

Rosemary

Myrtle

Thyme linalol

Basil linalol

Marjoram

Ginger

Other Care

Warmth often helps. For joints that feel painful, cold, and very stiff hold a covered hot water bottle over the area. For joints that are inflamed and hot to the touch: use a cold compress over the area. The herbal supplement cats claw can be very helpful, as can devil's claw. Regular swimming in warm water can help keep joints supple, as can other forms of gentle exercise.

When to Get Help

Consult your doctor if any of the following occur:

- The child has a high fever with pain and swelling in their joints or limbs. (Consult immediately.)
- The child has been injured, and the injury continues to be painful and sore and appears red or inflamed.
- The child appears to be limping or not using their joints properly.
- Morning stiffness, or if there are general aches and pain around the body.

ASTHMA

Asthma is caused by irritation in the breathing pathways to the lungs. The pathways become clogged with mucus and constrict so that breathing is difficult. According to the American Medical Association there are 5 million adult and child asthma sufferers in the U.S. today. Asthma can affect a person at any age, even babies. The attacks range in severity from very mild to life threatening. Some children outgrow asthma and stop having attacks around puberty. Asthma often runs in families, and more often occurs in families where there is a history of eczema, psoriasis, or hay fever.

There are many triggers to asthma attacks that differ from person to person. An attack might be brought on by an ear, nose, or throat infection, pollution in the atmosphere, house dust, pets, perfumes, and/or other commercial fragrance products. Some children may have allergies to medications or particular foods — or be sensitive to the preservatives or pesticides used in manufacturing them, including sulfates. Stress and anxiety are other factors that might be causing difficulties in breathing.

It's really worthwhile to try to establish which things might be triggers to your child's asthma attacks. Keep a diary and record each time your child has an attack, noting all things that happened at that time: what drink or foods were eaten, whether any medication was taken (both for the asthma and for other conditions), whether the child was inside or outside when the attack occurred, pollen conditions, pollution levels, emotional stress, anything surrounding the incident. Even ask yourself, "Did I spray air freshener or perfume before the attack?" As time goes on, you will build a record that will help enable you to identify some of the child's personal triggers.

Modern farming methods involve the addition of products that may be the cause of an attack. The growth hormone given to cows, which has been found in some milk, may cause a reaction in some children. Dairy products also cause the build up of mucus so try to cut down on dairy where possible if that seems to produce an attack. Wheat and other grains can be a trigger for asthma, especially if grown using pesticides, herbicides, or fungicides. Change to organic produce and see if that makes a difference. If not, cut wheat out of the diet altogether for a short period to see if there is any change. Go through all of the grains in this way, one after the other, and see if there is one acting as a trigger. Also, cut down on soda drinks.

Although pets are a delightful addition to a home, it is possible your child may be allergic to them. Compare your child's incidence of attacks while around animals and away from them. Also, be aware of your own moods. Many children take on the emotions of their parents/caretakers, so if you feel anxious, the child may too, and may have an attack because of it. Let your child be a child, unburdened by worries, for as long as you can, without mollycoddling them. Let them run free and exercise if they feel well enough to do so.

Signs and Symptoms

- wheezing with coughing
- coughing when trying to exhale; difficulty inhaling
- pains in the chest when breathing
- a feeling of constriction or tightness in the chest

The very fact of having an asthma attack can lead to a child feeling anxious. The following mixture of essential oils may help to calm your child, allowing a peaceful sleep. Also, having this calming bath before bed may prevent an anxiety-induced attack during the night.

Calming Bath Mix

First mix the following essential oils in 1 tablespoon of vegetable oil:

5 drops camomile roman
4 drops mandarin
1 drop geranium

Then add the following amount to a bath:

Use $^1/_4$ teaspoon if the child is 4 year old or under.
Use $^1/_2$ teaspoon if the child is between 5–8 years.
Use 1 teaspoon if the child is between 8–12 years.

Massage and Inhalation Mix

First make up a mix of essential oils using these proportions:

10 drops niaouli
4 drops marjoram
2 drops frankincense
10 drops camomile roman

Bottle the mix for future use.

Inhalation

One drop of the mix can be put on a tissue and inhaled when the child feels an attack may be coming, or if the child is under stress and you think they may have an attack.

Back and Chest Massage

To make a massage oil, take the following number of drops from the bottle, depending on the age of the child, and dilute in 1 teaspoon (5 ml.) of vegetable oil.

Age	Essential Oils
Up to 2 years	1 drop (use only a tiny amount each time)
2–5 years	2 drops in 1 teaspoon
5–8 years	3 drops in 1 teaspoon
8–11 years	4 drops in 1 teaspoon
12–16 years	5 drops in 1 teaspoon

Back massage may help reduce the frequency of asthma attacks. Massage over the whole back in large, sweeping movements in an upward direction. Also, massage the chest in the same way, more gently than the back. Use enough of the massage oil so the area is covered, but not so much that the skin remains oily. For children under 2 years of age, don't use the whole teaspoon of mix — just use a tiny amount.

Alternative Massage Mixes

Up to 2 years	2–7 years	7 years and over
Mix in 1 ounce vegetable oil: 5 drops lavender *or* 5 drops geranium	Mix in 1 ounce vegetable oil: 5 drops lavender 3 drops geranium 3 drops frankincense	Mix in 1 ounce vegetable oil: 5 drops geranium 5 drops cypress 5 drops frankincense

Essential Oils That Help

Lavender
Geranium
Frankincense
Cypress
Niaouli

Marjoram
Petitgrain
Camomile german
Camomile roman

Other Care

"Buteyko" is a breathing technique developed by a Russian doctor that has been helpful in cutting down the frequency of asthma attacks. Information is available on the internet under "buteyko," or see if your bookstore has anything on the subject.

Encourage your child to do The Cave Man Eating Plan, on page 40.

When to Get Help

Get immediate medical attention if your child does not respond to their regular prescribed medication.

Prevention

- Keep a diary of possible triggers.
- Let the child exercise.
- Try not to let the child become aware of your own stress.

ATHLETE'S FOOT

Athlete's foot, a fungal infection received its name because it's so often picked up by sporty types who spend a lot of time walking around communal locker rooms, showers, or swimming pools. It can also be transmitted by sharing footwear, towels, and bath mats. It's caused by the fungus *tinea,* and affects the area between the toes, the toenails, and the soles of the feet.

Signs and Symptoms
- soft, white, scaling skin; or dry, peeling skin; cracking, open flesh
- itching between toes, burning sensation, redness
- thickened, yellowing toenails
- foot odor
- possibly a rash resembling a group of small blisters

If your child catches athlete's foot, their feet should be kept as clean and dry as possible. Bathing the feet several times a day does help with the itching. This is obviously difficult to manage when the child is at school all day, so just do what you can.

Foot Bath and Dab	Foot Powder	Foot Massage Oil
Prepare the foot bath in a plastic bowl. Fill with warm water and add: 1 tablespoon bicarbonate of soda 1 tablespoon Epsom salts 2 tablespoons cider vinegar 5 drops tea tree Soak the feet for at least five minutes a day and dry them thoroughly. Then dab between the toes and around the toenails with the following concentrated essential oil mix using the tip of a cotton swab. 30 drops tea tree 30 drops manuka 2 drops cypress Use only a tiny smear each time.	Powder between the toes every day with a small amount of the following: 1 cup green clay 10 drops tea tree 10 drops manuka Mix the ingredients in a blender. Alternatively, just add the essential oils to the clay, while stirring fast. It will still go lumpy so wait for it to dry, then crunch the lumps into the rest of the clay and mix well.	Apply to the affected areas. Use a small amount of the following each time you massage the area: 1 tablespoon sesame oil 5 drops tea tree 1 drop lemon 3 drops manuka This is easiest to use at night, after the foot bath, and having dried the feet well.

Essential Oils That Help

There are essential oils that are appropriate for adult use but with children only the following are recommended:

Tea tree
Manuka
Lemongrass

Cypress
Palmarosa

When to Get Help

If the fungus appears to be spreading, seek professional advice. If, after three weeks of either pharmaceutical or home treatment, there is no improvement seek professional advice.

Prevention

- This fungus likes damp skin so always dry feet thoroughly. Sneakers are very comfortable and convenient, however, you many want to try other types of shoes at times. Don't let the child go barefoot, but they can wear open toe shoes around the house, and sandals when the weather permits.
- Choose natural fiber socks, preferably cotton. Use clean socks each day.
- Make sure shoes are thoroughly dry before wearing.
- Use antifungal preparations in both shoes after each wear, especially if other members of the household have athlete's foot.

ATTENTION DEFICIT DISORDERS (ADD)

A huge number of children in the United States have been diagnosed as having an attention deficit disorder (ADD), and many are on medication for it. ADD covers a wide range of characteristic behavior patterns relating to learning ability and social skills. As a society we should be concerned that so many of our children are experiencing these difficulties.

Figures show that ADD affects more boys than girls and seems to run in families. ADD includes a condition known as ADHD — attention deficit hyperactive disorder. Children under three years of age cannot be diagnosed with ADD or ADHD or put on medication for it because the symptoms of the disorder could be said to apply to all normal children of this age.

Signs and Symptoms

- poor attention span; easily distracted; difficulty in concentration
- disorganized and losing things frequently; learning difficulties
- difficulty following instructions; difficulty in accepting authority
- impulsive behavior; mood swings
- poor school performance
- ADHD — hyperactivity; sleeplessness; headaches

There are many other quite specific symptom indicators. These include shouting out the answer in class before being asked by the teacher, being disruptive in class, and not being able to wait patiently in line. Children can also engage in dangerous behavior, almost as if they have lost their sense of fear. This is what worries society so greatly — children out of control — and it perhaps explains why so many children are put on medication.

At present, there is no known specific cause of ADD, and it's likely there are many factors involved. Symptoms vary from child to child, and some may have developed the condition because of a nervous system disorder, dysfunctional brain development, brain injury, or having been born premature, or been a drug dependent baby. Other causes of ADD may be environmental, such as chemical farming methods and food additives, or industrial and vehicle pollution. It has even been suggested that ADD is caused by immunization.

Before worrying about all these things we need first to ask, does the child actually have attention deficit disorder? The symptoms listed above could be applied to many children who are going through the normal development process. All children get bored and frustrated, and act impulsively. One symptom of ADD is given as "not being able to play with one toy, but moving on to another." All children do this, and if some do it faster than others it is not surprising, given the type of society we live in. Think about television, with so many channels to choose from, we flick between them rapidly with the remote control. Children grow up with this, so it's not surprising if they think it's normal to change from one toy to another, as we flick between channels. If we want our children to concentrate on one thing at a time we have to give them the environment in which they can learn such a skill. There was a time when children spent hours pushing the same toy car around the floor. Now they have computers and zap monsters that move around in a split second. We need to spend time with our children and teach them to slow down.

Some characteristics of ADD could equally be applied to adults — making careless mistakes, not paying close attention to instructions, disrespect of authority, not finishing assignments because there is something else to do. Our children do not live in a vacuum, they watch and copy us.

Having said all that, for whatever reason, some children do have what might be diagnosed as ADD, and essential oils may be able to help them. All children have to wash, and essential oils can help make this a time of calming down, and soothing.

Soothing Baths and Showers

First in a small bottle mix the essential oils together in these proportions:

20 drops mandarin
10 drops lavender
10 drops camomile roman

Baths

Dilute the essential oil mix above in 1 teaspoon of vegetable oil, using these amounts:

Age	Essential Oils
3–5 years	2 drops
6–8 years	3 drops
8–11 years	5 drops

Add to the bath water and swish around before the child gets in.

Showers

Before taking a shower, after the right water temperature has been reached, put 4 drops of the essential oil mix above on a wash cloth or sponge and place it at the bottom of the shower cubicle. This will allow the oil to permeate the air through the steam.

Body Oil

You can apply body oil on younger children, but older children will probably want to apply any body oil on themselves, although getting them to remember to do it might be a challenge! Use a small amount each time. Massaging on the back is best for this condition.

Add the following essential oils to 2 ounces vegetable oil:

10 drops tangerine
5 drops cardamom
5 drops lavender

Helping Concentration

Studies have shown that essential oils can help with focus and concentration. Diffuse essential oils in the atmosphere, such as:

lemon   *bergamot*
grapefruit   *pine*

Helping Sleep

Studies have also shown that sleep is easier when essential oils are used. Lavender would be an excellent choice.

Diffuse it in the room before going to bed but not overnight. Or place a drop of lavender essential oil on the underside of the pillow, away from the eyes. It doesn't stain, and washes out easily. A child with ADD will need 4 drops, but if the child is on medication, use 2 only drops.

Essential Oils That Help

The following essential oils are easily available and they help to soothe and calm children of all ages:

Mandarin	Petitgrain
Tangerine	Ho-wood
Camomile roman	Lavender

Other Care

Certain components in food are thought to make hyperactivity worse. Try to persuade your child to do The Cave Man Eating Plan on page 40, or at least cut down on the caffeine in sodas, sugar in general, and processed foods. Avoid food coloring wherever you can.

Find time to talk to your child and time to play together. Younger children can be discouraged from spending time watching television and sitting in front of the computer. See also: Computer-Related Disorders.

When to Get Help

Correct diagnosis is very important, and before medication is given you should get a second professional opinion. Your child may just be at a hyperactive stage of development. The symptoms of ADD may also be an expression of your child's frustration at having an undiagnosed learning difficulty such as dyslexia. Try to remember that most children go through a stage of hyperactivity at some time in their lives, sometimes only briefly. Above all, ensure your child is not just seeking your attention, because they feel they have too little of it. Time spent with a child playing outside games, indoor board games, or reading to each other pays great dividends in terms of good behavior and building a close relationship.

Prevention

- Assess for learning difficulty.
- Change diet.
- Do activities with child.
- Create a soothing atmosphere in the home.

BALANITIS

This rather scientific name, *balanitis,* means inflammation of the penis head, the glans. It can be caused by several things, including bacteria, fungi, wearing tight clothes, or having an allergy to the chemicals in diapers or clothes. Diaper rash can also cause it. Balanitis is more likely in boys who are not circumcised.

Signs and Symptoms
- penis is inflamed and sore on tip, or under and around foreskin
- if child is in diapers, buttocks and genital area may also be infected
- penis is swollen
- it is difficult to draw back the foreskin for cleaning

Bathing	Ointment
For babies up to 2 years of age, follow the directions for Diaper Rash.	For babies up to 2 years of age, follow the directions for Diaper Rash.
Essential oils in the bath ease irritation and discomfort. Blend the essential oils together, then for children 2–4 years old use 3 drops of the mix in the bath, for children 5–10 years old use between 4–5 drops in the bath. Mix together:	Apply a small amount of the ointment as needed:
1 teaspoon vegetable oil 3 drops camomile german 2 drops tea tree 1 drop palmarosa	$^1/_2$ ounce aloe vera gel $^1/_2$ ounce calendula infused oil 10 drops jojoba oil 10 drops lavender 6 drops geranium

Essential Oils That Help

Lavender	Manuka
Camomile german	Thyme linalol
Tea tree	Palmarosa

Other Care

Ensure the child bathes regularly, drawing back the foreskin gently to clean the area. Dry the penis thoroughly after every diaper change, or tell older children to dry themselves. Then apply the ointment.

If you suspect your laundry powder has caused an allergic reaction in your child, rinse and dry clothes already laundered and change your washing powder with the next wash.

When to Get Help

If an infection appears, or there is pus from the penis, tell your doctor. If the condition does not improve after a few days of home treatment, whether using a natural or pharmaceutical treatment, seek further help from your physician.

Prevention

- Ensure good hygiene.
- Check washing products are not causing an allergic reaction.
- Don't let child wear underpants or diapers that are too tight.

BITES — ANIMALS AND INSECTS

Children come into contact with all kinds of animals, both domestic and wild. Animal bites can be extremely dangerous and should always be seen by a physician or hospital as soon as possible. A tetanus injection may be needed, if the child's inoculation has not been kept up-to-date. This section offers immediate self-help advice on animal, snake, and insect bites, that can be carried out while waiting for further professional help.

Essential Oils That Help

Thyme	Camomile german
Oregano	Manuka
Eucalyptus radiata	Lemongrass
Ravensara	Geranium
Lavender	

Animal Bites

Wash the area of the bite with water and mild soap and then rinse with water and disinfectant. If the area is easily accessible, rinse in water running gently from a faucet for several minutes. Then dry and cover. If the wound is bleeding, apply pressure to the area with a clean piece of cloth, and make sure further help for the child is being arranged.

Rabies is a worry, especially where wildlife is concerned, although superficial wounds are not as risky as those that puncture the skin. If the skin is broken at all, or there is bleeding, or more than one bite, call your doctor or 911 immediately. Even if the skin was not broken at the time, if it starts to look red and swollen later, or infected under the surface, get immediate medical help.

Snake Bites

Try to keep the child and yourself calm and arrange for emergency medical help immediately. The bitten area should be kept as still as possible, so try to avoid unnecessary movement. While getting help, cover the bite with a cold compress on which you have put at least 25 drops of lavender oil. If you don't have any lavender to hand, use what you have, any essential oil is better than nothing at this point.

It's difficult to know whether the bite is poisonous or not, so just err on the side of caution and assume it is. It's highly likely the bite was poisonous if the fang marks are deep and prominent, or if any of the following symptoms occur.

Signs and Symptoms

- there is swelling, redness, bluishness, or a burning sensation around the area of bite
- the tissue around bite, as well as bite area itself, is very painful
- feeling faint, nausea, vomiting
- clammy skin; sweating
- rapid or too shallow breathing
- fast heart and pulse rate

Insect Bites

Insect bites cause pain, soreness, itching, swelling, and redness. Whatever the insect, get help if the child develops a rash or if the bite looks infected. If the child has difficulty in breathing, call emergency services immediately.

Allergic reaction to insect bites is common and signs may appear over the following 12 to 24 hours. Look for increased swelling in the area, redness, or hives. If any of these occur, or if the child is in pain, has breathing difficulties, nausea, or headache, get immediate medical attention.

Most insect bites can be soothed by applying a cold, wet compress on which 5 drops each of camomile german and lavender have been put. For more specific information see following pages.

Spiders

Mix the following together and apply a small amount to the area three times over the next 24 hours, or longer if needed:

1 teaspoon alcohol
3 drops lavender
2 drops camomile german

The black widow spider bite is particularly nasty, and is one that requires immediate medical attention. On your way to the doctor, apply 10 drops of neat lavender oil directly onto the bite every five minutes until you arrive.

Mosquitoes

Prevention is best where mosquitoes are concerned and they can be deterred by the smell of lavender. Put drops of neat lavender on clothing: socks, cloth shoes, collars, sleeves, and the bottom of skirts or trousers legs. At night, put lavender on tissues or cotton wool and tuck under the pillow or put on the bedside table. Other oils which help keep mosquitoes away are lemongrass, citronella, and eucalyptus citriodora.

For single bites:

Put 1 drop neat lavender oil directly on the bite.

For multiple bites, mix:

1 cup cider vinegar (or the juice of 2 lemons)
10 drops lavender
5 drops thyme linalol

Put the mixture in the bath, swishing the water around before putting the child in. Afterward, put neat lavender on the bites.

Gnat and Midge Bites

To stop the irritation, mix the following and apply over the whole affected area:

1 teaspoon cider vinegar (or lemon juice)
3 drops thyme linalol
1 tablespoon lavender hydrolat (or plain water)

Alternatively, apply neat lavender to the bites.

Bee Stings

Bee stings can cause fever and headaches, and if there's an allergic reaction there can be swelling, redness, and rash.

Try to remove the sting. Put a few drops of camomile german on a cold cider vinegar compress and apply to the area. If the position of the bite allows, leave the compress there for a couple of hours, otherwise for as long as possible. Then apply 1 drop of neat camomile german to the bite, 3 times a day for 2 days.

The following remedy for wasp stings can also be used.

Wasp Stings

Mix the following and dab onto the bitten area 3 times a day:

1 teaspoon cider (or wine) vinegar
2 drops lavender
2 drops camomile german

BLISTERS

Although the most common type of blister is the one caused by the shoe rubbing on the skin, there are other, more serious varieties. Blisters can form anywhere on the body due to an allergy, or viral or bacterial infection. For blisters cause by burns, see Burns and Sunburn.

Signs and Symptoms

- raised, thin skin filled with fluid, redness surrounding
- sore if pressed

Blisters on the Feet

Blisters form as a protection to stop further damage to tissue. They generally clear up by themselves over time. See Other Care, below.

If the skin is not broken apply a drop of the following neat essential oils:

lavender or lemon

Recycle those old tea bags! Put 1 drop geranium on a wet tea bag (black or green tea) and hold it over the blister.

If your child plays a lot of sports or is always wearing sport shoes and has repeated trouble with blisters, it may be worth toughening up their feet.

Mix the following together well and soak the feet for ten minutes at least once a week:

1 bowl of cold tea
1 tablespoon Epsom salts
1 drop myrrh essential oil diluted in 1 drop iodine

Blisters on the Body

Blisters on the body are a sign of infection or another problem that requires medical help. In the meantime, to help reduce the inflammation and pain, make up the hydrolat mix below, put in a new and clean plant mister and spray over the affected area.

equal parts lavender, camomile, and rose hydrolat
3 drops camomile roman
3 drops eucalyptus radiata

Shake well before use.

Essential Oils That Help

Tea tree	Lavender
Lemon	Camomile roman
Calendula (infused or absolute)	

Other Care

Always leave the blister as it is; and never try to get the fluid out while the skin underneath is in the process of healing. Leave the blistered area uncovered as much as possible so it has a chance to dry out and heal.

When to Get Help

Always consult a doctor if there are blisters on the body, if the child has a fever, or has blisters due to an allergy or from taking medication. Also, get further help if the blisters become infected, or have increased redness around the outer edges, or there is swelling.

Prevention

- Wear shoes that fit properly.
- Wear socks with sport shoes and closed leather shoes.
- At the first sign of redness protect heels or sore patches of the foot with blister dressings or Band-Aids.

BODY PIERCING

Today, body piercing appeals even to young children, who often find that a professional body-piercer will not carry out the work on them without their parent's consent. Consequently, children sometimes attempt their own body-piercing, or do it for their friends. However it is carried out, body piercing often results in soreness, infection, and inflammation.

The area is infected if it is red, swollen, feels raw, and/or there is a discharge. The discharge often dries into a crust around the ring or other pierced object, and around the immediate area. If this occurs, the pierced object should be removed. Earrings can be removed easily but any other body piercing should be removed professionally.

Infection occurs when bacteria gets into the wounded area. It's vital that the area be kept clean at all times to prevent infection. Pierced ears are at risk of infection from nearby hair, touching by fingers, and bed linen. If the piercing is covered by clothing, be sure it is covered with a sterile dressing. Otherwise, expose the area as much as possible because light and air assist in the healing process. Body piercings are prone to repeat infection. Infections can cause scar tissue under the surface of the skin and scarring on the surface.

Immediate Preventative Care

Prevention is best, so if your child has just had a body piercing, to help prevent infection, get a bowl of water and add 2 tablespoons salt to each pint of water. Bathe the pierced area with this salted water. Then put one drop neat tea tree over the pierced area.

Sore Holes (anywhere on the body)	Infected Holes (anywhere on the body)	In the Mouth
Add these essential oils to ¹/₂ ounce alcohol: 5 drops tea tree 5 drops geranium Add all this to a bowl of salt water and bathe the affected area/s.	First remove the pierced object. Clean the area at least 4 times a day with the alcohol mix in Sore Holes. Then use one drop of the following mix of essential oils over the affected area: 8 drops thyme linalol 5 drops ravensara 6 drops lavender 7 drops tea tree Do not use on mucous membrane areas.	Rinse the mouth out at least five times a day with the following, then spit it out. **Never swallow essential oils.** Add these essential oils to 1 ounce alcohol: 10 drops myrrh 2 drops frankincense 3 drops clove Blend together well, and bottle. For each mouth rinse, use 10 drops of this mix, added to a small glass of water.

Essential Oils That Help

Thyme linalol   Frankincense
Clove   Ravensara
Tea Tree   Niaouli
Myrrh
(Lavender may assist in closing the hole)

Other Care

Tincture of myrrh may be used for mouth or tongue piercings only.

BOILS

A boil is a skin infection usually caused by the bacteria *staphylococci*. The boil forms into a pus-filled lumpy area under the surface of the skin and is very sore and painful. It shouldn't be confused with a pus-filled spot, which is near the surface of the skin (see Acne). Children of all ages can develop boils, whether babies or teenagers. Boils can appear on all areas, particularly the buttocks, face, nose, neck, ears, back, armpits, and groin. Infection in a hair follicle can often result in a boil.

Signs and Symptoms
- sore and painful red lump under surface of skin that becomes harder over time
- can be soreness around area
- can have swollen lymph glands

Washing	Hot Compresses and Oil Method
Bathe the area twice a day with the following essential oils put in a small bowl of hot water and swished around: 2 drops lavender 2 drops tea tree If the inflammation is severe add: 1 drop camomile	To draw out the pus, put 1 drop of red thyme on a hot compress and apply fresh twice a day. When the pus has come out, apply a small amount of the following mix over the area, twice a day: 1 teaspoon vegetable oil 3 drops lavender 2 drops thyme linalol 2 drops tea tree

While pus is coming out of the boil it's extremely important to keep the area as clean as possible and change dressings frequently. Be careful no pus gets on any other part of the body as this may cause further infection and boils. Epsom salts and sea salt are effective additions to water when cleansing the area. If the boil is on a buttock, a bowl can be filled with a washing solution and sat in. This might look and feel comical but it does bring relief.

While Pus Is Coming Out

Cleansing Soak	Compresses
This mix can be used to soak the area of the boil. If the area cannot be soaked, use this to wash the area as often as possible. Swish around to disperse oils before use: 2 pints water 1 teaspoon Epsom salts 1 teaspoon sea salt 2 drops lavender 2 drops tea tree 1 drop thyme linalol Larger quantities can be made using these proportions.	To draw out the pus: make the cleansing soak mix using hot water, then soak a clean piece of light-weight natural material (muslin is ideal) in the hot mixture, squeeze out, and hold over the boil until cool. Repeat 3 times. Then cover the boil with a dressing on which you've put 1 drop lemon and 1 drop lavender. The part of the dressing with the essential oils should be directly over the boil.

Essential Oils That Help

Lavender   Tea tree
Manuka   Lemon
Thyme linalol   Eucalyptus radiata

Other Care

Treat boils as an infection and do not share towels, wash cloths, etc. Do not squeeze boils, they will eventually come to a head and burst. Keep the area covered to prevent further infection and change dressings frequently. If the boil is on an area that gets rubbed by clothes, apply an extra large, thick dressing to make it less sore. If the boil is on a baby's buttocks, change diapers more frequently and, whenever possible, expose the skin to the air.

When to Get Help

It is vital that you get immediate medical help if you notice a thin red line running in the direction of the heart, away from the boil — to the neck, armpit, or groin. This may be caused by the infection spreading through the blood stream to other areas of the body.

Continuously getting boils may indicate there is another disorder present and a doctor's advice should be sought. Also, contact your doctor if there is more than one boil and they seem to be multiplying, the child feels ill or has a fever, or if the infection does not clear up after the boil has discharged all the pus. Boils sometimes need to be lanced, and this should never be done at home. Lancing a boil should always be done by a qualified medical practitioner.

Prevention

- Keep body hair areas scrupulously clean as boils often appear where bacteria has entered the hair follicle as a result of the action of clothes rubbing that area.

BROKEN BONES AND FRACTURES

Bones can be broken, splintered, displaced, or dislocated at the joint. The only way to know the exact nature of the damage is to get an X ray and immediate medical attention. Hair line fractures in small children may only need to be in plaster for a few days. Children's bones are more pliable than adults' and sometimes bend rather than break.

Although a broken bone needs to be set in plaster as soon as possible, home assistance can help the mind and body cope with the trauma, so that all the body's healing energy is focused on repairing the fracture as quickly as possible.

Signs and Symptoms

- pain
- swelling
- lack of mobility

To Ease the Trauma	To Help Speed Healing
To help with the pain and to calm the child, put a few drops of lavender essential oil near the break and spread very gently around.	After the bone has been set in plaster essential oils can be put on the exposed surrounding skin. Take care not to move or dislodge the bone. Simply smooth the mix on the available skin; do not massage or rub in. The following mix can be used on children over 5 years of age. Use a small amount only with each application: 1 ounce St. John's Wort infused oil 10 drops ginger 5 drops lavender 2 drops helichrysum (also known as Italian everlasting or immortelle)

Essential Oils That Help

Lavender	Myrtle
Ginger	Spikenard
Camomile roman	Helichrysum
St. John's Wort infused oil	
Calendula infused oil	

Other Care

Cold compresses may help ease the pain while waiting for medical help. These can be made using cold water, witch hazel, or a solution of water and the essential oils listed above. Homeopathic arnica tablets can also be given, as well as Dr. Bach's Rescue Remedy.

When to Get Help

Get emergency medical help immediately.

BRONCHIOLITIS

For children over 2 years of age, see also Bronchitis

Bronchiolitis is an infection of the air tubes, the bronchioles, mostly affecting babies and children under 2 years of age. The infection is usually viral (such as *respiratory syncytial virus*). It results in inflammation and narrowing of the air tubes along with a build up of mucus.

The infection is easily spread in the air, and can even contaminate surfaces that are then touched by a young child. As it's more usual in the colder months, the first symptoms are often mistaken for the common cold. Antibiotics are not usually effective against this type of virus while essential oils can be highly useful.

Keep the child warm, cozy, and calm by offering them lots of attention. Give plenty of liquids, and feed them in frequent small amounts, rather than infrequent large amounts.

Signs and Symptoms

- runny nose, sniffles, sneezing, coughing
- unable to breathe properly, rapid breathing, shallow breaths, wheezing
- temperature, fever, feeling generally unwell
- refuses food and fluids
- sometimes lips and mouth seem bluish
- can be mistaken for the common cold

Bronchiolitis Mix

The following mix can be used in three ways. Make up a batch using these proportions and bottle:

20 drops niaouli
10 drops ravensara
8 drops thyme linalol

Room Steamer	Drops on Material	Massage
Put the essential oils into a bowl of steaming hot water and place in the same room as baby, out of reach of children and pets. Use these amounts: up to 1 year 5 drops over 1 year 8 drops	To help breathing during the night put 2 drops of the Bronchiolitis mix on the back of the child's night clothes and on a corner of a pillow or mattress cover, somewhere away from the eyes.	Use 5 drops of the Bronchiolitis mix in 1 teaspoon almond oil. With children under 2 years of age, rub a small amount of this over the back of their body. Imagine where their lungs are, and apply on that area on the back. Do this twice a day. For children over 2 years old, before applying the oil, put 2 drops of the mix directly on your hands, rub them together, and wipe over the child's front and back. Then apply a small amount of the massage oil over the back, as above.

Essential Oils That Help Fight the Infection

Niaouli
Ravensara
Eucalyptus radiata
Thyme linalol
Myrtle

Essential Oils That Help Keep the Child Calm

Lavender
Camomile roman
Mandarin
Can be diluted and massaged into the feet

Other Care

Give your child plenty of fluids to drink. Liquids will soothe them and help to prevent them from becoming distressed which makes breathing more difficult. The American Medical Association recommends that a humidifier is used in the child's room and essential oils can be added to them. Essential oil mist vaporizers or sprays are also helpful.

When to Get Help

As soon as the child develops cold-like symptoms, keep a close eye on them to make sure the infection does not worsen. If it does, seek medical attention as the child may need oxygen to enable them to breathe properly. Hospitalization may be required.

Prevention

- Keep babies and young children away from anyone who is sneezing or shows signs of having a cold or flu.
- If someone living in the home has a cold or flu, diffuse essential oils from the fight infection list of oils above, throughout the house to help keep it from being passed on.
- If someone traveling in the same car as the baby has a cold or flu, put one drop of essential oil, from the fight infection list on a tissue and tuck near baby's seat.

BRONCHITIS

Bronchitis is an inflammation of the membranes lining the airways or bronchial tubes. It is usually a complication of a viral or bacterial infection that often starts with cold or flu type symptoms — runny nose, sniffles, sore throat, developing into a deep, chesty cough. The inflammation can be made worse by a smoky or polluted atmosphere.

Keep the child as calm and stress-free as possible. It's better that the phlegm is released through cough than held in. Try to get the child to spit phlegm out. See Other Care, below.

Signs and Symptoms

- dry cough or mucus cough, feels sore when child coughs
- yellow phlegm
- wheezing, chest pain
- fever

Bronchitis Mix		
The following mix can be used in three ways. Make up a batch using these proportions and bottle: 10 drops thyme linalol 10 drops eucalyptus radiata 10 drops niaouli 25 drops myrtle		
Room Steamer	**Tissue**	**Massage**
Put 10 drops of the bronchitis mix into a bowl of steaming hot water and place in the same room as the child, but out of reach of all children and pets.	To help breathing during the night, put 4 drops on a tissue and tuck near the child's head, away from their eyes.	Use 3–5 drops of the above mix in a teaspoon of vegetable oil and massage a small amount over the chest and back of the child.

Essential Oils That Help

Niaouli   Ravensara
Myrtle   Thyme linalol
Eucalyptus radiata
Bronchodect (see Suppliers)

Other Care

The American Medical Association recommends humidifiers or steam to help keep the bronchial passages clear. Both methods can be used with essential oils. If the child is coughing, to encourage the release of phlegm, hold them over your lap, face down. Keep the child's head propped up at night. Have them drink plenty of liquid and eat frequent small meals rather than infrequent large ones.

When to Get Help

There can be complications with bronchitis so always get a diagnosis and be prepared to contact help again if the condition gets worse, or if it doesn't seem to be getting better. Get immediate help if the child is wheezing, vomiting, or has a bluish tinge around the lips and mouth.

Prevention

- Same as for Bronchiolitis.

BURNS

No matter how vigilant we are, children get themselves into accidents. That is the nature of children — they like to explore and move about, and sometimes they get burned. As well as by fire, children are burned by hot objects, hot liquids, steam, electricity, radiation, and chemicals. Electrical burns are often worse than they look, so get an immediate medical opinion on them. Shock is a danger with all burns and it may come on hours after the event. It's always better to be on the safe side and get a professional opinion.

Signs and Symptoms

- *First Degree or Superficial Burns*
  There is a red area or patch of skin over which a blister might form, filled with a water-like substance. Only small burns of this type can be treated with the following suggestions.

- *Second Degree Burns*
  There is a great deal of pain, redness, swelling, or blistering. Immediate emergency medical treatment must be sought.

- *Third Degree Burns*
  These burns affect the deeper tissue of the body and are very dangerous. The skin may appear brown or black instead of red, and because the nerve endings are damaged, there may not be any pain. Immediate emergency medical treatment must be sought.

First Action — All Burns

Cool the skin by immersing in cold water — the colder the better. Do not use ice. The water could be from a faucet at a sink, bath, or shower — whatever cold water source is closest. Adjust the tap until the water is flowing gently. Put the burned area into the flow, and keep the child as still as possible until the burned area cools down, approximately 10 minutes. You could also use water in a bowl, set inside a larger bowl filled with ice to keep it cool. If the skin is intact, add a few drops of lavender oil on the cold water and swish it around.

If the burn appears to be anything more than superficial immediately arrange for medical help.

Second Action — Home Treatment

Oil should never be placed on a burn, however, essential oils are not oily as such, and providing the skin is not blistered or broken, can be applied, but only after all the first-aid cooling measures have been taken. Essential oils became known for their use on burns after lavender was used on burns in the early 1900s after a laboratory accident. That accident has become part of modern aromatherapy history.

a) If no broken skin or broken blisters:
Put 2 drops neat lavender oil directly on the area of the burn.

b) If the skin is broken or the blister is broken:
Put 2 drops neat lavender oil around the area of the burn.

All cases:
Then put 5 drops lavender on a dry, cold compress, and use it to cover the area.

Repeat a) or b) and compress, as needed.

Heat Burns	Chemical Burns
Apply a cold compress.	*Cover the area with a clean dressing. Get to an emergency department immediately if a lower layer of skin has been exposed, or if there are signs of infection, or damage other than redness.*

Essential Oils That Help

Lavender
Camomile german

Other Care

Cover the burned area with clean, non-fluffy, material. Don't apply any greasy substances such as butter, margarine, or vegetable oil. Give the child lots of cool drinks, and keep their body warm.

When to Get Help

Remember that with burns there is a danger of your child going into shock (see Shock). Always call your doctor if the burn is from a chemical or electrical source, even if the burn appears to be superficial.

In the case of other burns, get medical attention if it does not appear to be healing, if it becomes more red or swollen, or it develops areas of pus.

Prevention

- Keep your child away from fire, matches, and cigarettes.
- Check that dangerous chemicals and other liquids are out of reach of children.
- Check that electrical equipment and wiring is out of reach, and that wall sockets are fitted with child-protection covers.

CATARRH

When a child has too much mucus in their throat and nose it's called catarrh. It's one of the body's self-defense mechanisms, as it produces mucus to try and rid the body of bacteria, viruses, and other irritants. Catarrh usually accompanies or follows conditions that affect the respiratory system, such as colds, flu, hay fever, sinusitis, even measles, and ear infections.

Signs and Symptoms
- stuffy nose; unable to breathe easily
- runny nose
- coughing

Humidifier	Chest Rub
Add to the water in the humidifier:	The following mix will help clear a congested chest.
4 drops ravensara 2 drops eucalyptus radiata	Apply a small amount on the chest and back, before bedtime.
If the inflammation is severe add:	
1 drop camomile	

Steaming Bowl Inhalation Method
This method should only be used with children old enough to understand why they should keep their hands off the table and out of the way of the hot water. To a small bowl of steaming water, add: 4 drops eucalyptus radiata alternatively, use menthol crystals Your child should inhale the aromatic steam through their nose. Make sure they keep their mouth and eyes shut. Put a towel over the child's head — big enough to hang down to the shoulders — to stop the steam from escaping. Use this method once a day for two to five days.

Essential Oils That Help

Ravensara	Elemi
Eucalyptus radiata	Frankincense
Niaouli	

Other Care

Breathing at night can be made easier if you prop your child up against pillows. Give your child plenty of drinks, especially water. Get your child to blow their nose and clear their throat, rather than sniffing the mucus back up.

When to Get Help

With babies, get help if the catarrh is making feeding difficult, or if you think the baby's catarrh is due to an allergy. Also, seek medical advice if your child has an ear infection that may be causing the catarrh.

CHICKENPOX

Chickenpox is a contagious viral infection that can only be caught by being in direct contact with a person who has either chickenpox or shingles — the adult version of the infection. Chickenpox spreads very easily from child to child, and although it's said a child's immunity to it is built up after having it once, the fact is some children have chickenpox 2 or 3 times during their childhood years.

Children with weakened immune systems can have the disease far more seriously than those with healthy immune systems. Chickenpox affects children of all ages. It's important the child doesn't scratch the scabs as they can become infected and leave scars.

To help prevent other people in the household from catching chickenpox, spray the atmosphere with antiviral essential oils (see Antiinfectious Air Spray page 37).

Signs and Symptoms

- *First Sign:* mild fever, feeling unwell and/or cranky, headache, chills
- *Second Sign:* a rash of small red spots on the child's body and scalp turning to:
- *Third Sign:* fluid-filled blisters, that cause intense itching turning to:
- *Last Sign:* scabs that eventually drop off

Baths

If a child is calm, they will sleep better and scratch less. All the following bath methods will help induce calm and sleep.

Oat Bath	Salt Bath	Soothing Bath
Put a handful of oatmeal or raw oats into a piece of material and close securely. Drop the following essential oils onto the material: 4 drops camomile german 4 drops lavender Attach the bundle to the faucet, or hold there, so the water gently runs through it before reaching the bath.	When the water has been run, add a tablespoon of sea salt to the bath plus: 1 drop lavender 1 drop tea tree	Into 1 cup of baking soda add: 2 drops lavender 1 drop camomile german Mix well with a spoon before adding to the bath water.

Diffuser Mix to Aid Sleep

Use the following essential oils in a diffuser or spray to help induce sleep:

2 drops lavender
4 drops petitgrain

Anti-Itching Lotion

This lotion can be dabbed onto the spots after baths, or when needed.
Dab on the spots, allow to dry, then repeat.

Be careful to keep the lotion away from the eyes. Mix together:
2 ounces lavender hydrolat/water
2 ounces camomile hydrolat/water
4 drops lavender
4 drops camomile german
2 drops eucalyptus radiata
2 drops ravensara

Shake the ingredients together in a bottle. The essential oils will still float on the surface. Continue to shake vigorously, then pour through an unbleached paper coffee filter into a measuring jug and rebottle.

Calamine Lotion and Essential Oil Mix

To an 8-ounce bottle of calamine lotion add:

10 drops camomile german
30 drops lavender

Shake well and apply to affected areas of skin.

Essential Oils That Help

Lavender
Camomile german
Camomile roman

Other Care

Calamine lotion is the traditionally used, soothing preparation for this condition. Spread it over the affected area and leave for a few hours or overnight. The American Medical Association recommends soothing baths, and essential oils can be added to vegetable oil and then put in the water. Swish it all around well before the child gets in.

If blisters are in the throat, have the child gargle with salt water that has had a small amount of vinegar and honey added.

When to Get Help

It is wise to get a doctor's diagnosis as soon as possible and call the doctor again if the child has any swelling, develops a cough, or sore throat.

Prevention

With most children starting child care at a very early age, it is very difficult to prevent a child from getting chickenpox. To keep a child from spreading chickenpox, keep them at home until your doctor tells you they are no longer contagious.

Children with chickenpox should be kept away from adults who have never had the infection. This is because, when infected for the first time in adulthood, shingles can develop, which is a more serious and recurring problem.

CIRCUMCISION

Circumcision is not a condition, but a procedure.

For boys, it's the surgical removal of the foreskin, carried out under local anaesthetic. The inner and outer layers of the foreskin are removed, there are a few stitches, and a dressing is applied. Circumcision may be carried out for medical reasons, perhaps the foreskin is too tight, or there are hygiene factors. More usually, it is a religious ritual of both the Jewish and Muslim traditions, sometimes performed by a rabbi or religious leader. In some groups it is performed shortly after birth, while in others, either before or at puberty — when the boy is often given fabulous clothes to wear, and receives gifts of money from relatives and friends.

For girls, circumcision is altogether different. In some countries, girls between 8 and 12 years of age are cut around the genital area. Often with no anaesthetic or medical assistance, a traditional tribal healer, or local woman practicing female circumcision will remove some or all of the clitoris, also possibly the labia, minora, and majora, and at times narrow the entrance to the vagina with stitches.

Female circumcision has no religious involvement (or basis in religious writings). It's the women of the community, including the mothers and grandmothers, who insist on continuing the practice. They believe girls will not be able to find a husband if they can't prove, by circumcision, that their sexuality is under control and their fidelity assured.

In 1980 it was estimated that 84 million women, in 30 African countries, had been circumcised. Today, many African mothers bring their daughters to the West in order to avoid having their daughter endure the procedure. Although female circumcision is illegal in Western countries, the tradition is still so strong that some doctors of the same culture practicing in the West, clandestinely perform the procedure, when there is no valid medical or hygienic reason for it. Complications can arise from these less professionally carried out cases.

Complications of the Procedure
- infection
- redness, pain, swelling, pus

Infection Prevention for Boys

First, prepare the antiseptic wash or spray for the area.

In 1 pint of warm water add 20 drops of lavender essential oil.

Bottle, and shake very well. Now pour through a paper coffee filter, and rebottle. Use before circumcision — as a rinse after washing, or in a spray, over the genital area. Use after circumcision to also assist in healing, once the dressing has been removed.

Sitz Baths for Boys and Girls

In a large plastic bowl full of warm water, add:

1 teaspoon salt
7 drops lavender

Swish the water around well. Your child should sit in this sitz bath for approximately 10 minutes or so.

Compresses for Boys and Girls

Use the compress method made with:

lavender hydrolat
camomile hydrolat

Use one single hydrolat or combine them. Use a soft, muslin-type material folded over a few times. Soak it in the hydrolat, squeeze out well, and apply to the genitals.

Calming Back Rub for Girls

Make a calming body rub by mixing the following:

1 ounce vegetable oil
5 drops geranium
5 drops rose otto

Use a small amount each time to rub over your child's back.

Shock for Girls

Refer to the Shock section.

Essential Oils That Help

Lavender   Geranium

Camomile   Rose otto

Other Care

Use whatever traditional healing medicine is given in these circumstances, providing you know it is effective.

When to Get Help

In both boys and girls get immediate medical help if there is any sign of infection.

If, because of cultural pressure, circumcision has been carried out on your daughter, recently or in the past, legally or illegally, please seek professional medical care as soon as possible.

COLDS (THE COMMON COLD)

Colds are perhaps the most common ailment for both children and adults. They are an infection by various types of viruses, all contagious. A child of any age can catch a cold, but it's especially distressing for babies who experience difficulty drinking from a bottle or the breast when they have a stuffed-up nose.

Antibiotics cannot treat colds and are best avoided at this time. A child's tolerance to antibiotics can build up if they are taken too frequently. A child may then require a higher dose of an antibiotic, and in some cases, a child can build up a resistance to certain antibiotics if taken too frequently.

Signs and Symptoms

- runny nose, stuffed nose
- congestion — often in the chest
- cough
- fever

The Colds Mix

This blend of essential oils can be used in a variety of methods.

Mix the oils in these proportions and bottle for when needed:

10 drops eucalyptus radiata
10 drops ravensara
5 drops tea tree
3 drops lavender
1 drop thyme linalol

Baths	**Tissue**

Dilute the colds mix in vegetable oil before adding it to a bath. Use these amounts, depending on the age of the child:
 	
babies 2–18 months   1 drop of colds mix in
                            1 teaspoon vegetable oil
 	
18 months–3 years   2 drops of colds mix in
                            1 teaspoon vegetable oil
 	
3–6 years   3 drops of colds mix in
                            1 teaspoon vegetable oil
 	
7–11 years   4 drops of colds mix in
                            1 teaspoon vegetable oil
 	
12 years old and over   5 drops of colds mix in
                            1 teaspoon vegetable oil
 	
For babies under 2 months, put 1 drop of the colds mix in 2 teaspoons vegetable oil, blend well, and use only $1/2$ teaspoon per bath.
	Put 2 drops of the colds mix on a tissue. The child can sniff from this to help relieve the symptoms.

Inhalation	**Steam Method**	**Baby Massage**
This method should only be used by children who are old enough to understand the danger of hot water. See Inhalation Method on page 20 for directions. Use 3 drops of the colds mix per inhalation.	This method is effective with babies. See Water Bowl Method on page 22 for directions. Place the bowl of steaming water near or under the crib or bed. Add to it: 3 drops of colds mix	Massage into the upper chest and back at each diaper change: 2 teaspoons vegetable oil 1 drop colds mix Only use a very tiny amount of the mix each time.

Sinus Massage

This can only be used on children over 3 years of age.

Smooth a tiny amount of the following mix over the nose, sinus area of the upper cheek, and above the eyebrows. Use very little at a time, being careful the oil does not go near the eyes, and wipe any excess off with a tissue. This can be done after the child has fallen asleep. Use only a very small amount of this mix with each application:

1 tablespoon vegetable oil
2 drops lemon
1 drop niaouli
5 drops colds mix

Foot Massage for Chills

If the child has a chill that makes them feel cold and shivery, massage both feet with the following mix before bedtime.

1 teaspoon vegetable oil
1 drop ginger
1 drop ormenis flower (camomile maroc)

Ensure the child has adequate bedclothes.

Essential Oils That Help

Tea tree
Thyme linalol
Ravensara

Eucalyptus radiata
Manuka
Niaouli

Other Care

Keep your child warm, snug, and calm. Fresh air is a far better atmosphere for the child than virus-laden warm air, so open the windows when your child leaves a room to keep the home healthily ventilated. Use a mix of Antiinfectious Air Spray in a diffuser (see list on page 37). Have your child drink plenty of fluids, especially water.

When to Get Help

Get medical advice if your child has a temperature over 102 degrees or if they complain of earache and neck pain, or if their difficult breathing does not seem to improve.

Prevention

- Keep babies away from people who have colds or are sneezing.
- Colds very often pass from person to person within the home. Spray rooms frequently with Antiinfectious Air Spray (see pages 37 for method, and pages 34–35 for list of oils); and ask any person in the home with a cold to keep away from the children as much as possible until the cold has passed.
- If colds are going around your child's school, send them with a tissue on which you have put 2 drops of the colds mix. The child can sniff from this during the day. Tell other mothers, fathers, and caretakers what you are doing, as they might want to join you in this preventative measure.

COLD SORES (FEVER BLISTERS)

Cold sores are caused by the virus, herpes simplex 1. They're caught by kissing someone who is infected, by sharing cups and utensils, or by some other contact. There may not be an outbreak of blisters with the initial infection, and the child may just have flu like symptoms. Once caught, however, the cold sore virus will be with the child for their lifetime. According to the American Medical Association most affected people had their initial infection when they were between the ages of 6 months and 5 years old.

The virus lives permanently on the nerve-ending where initial contact was made. It may be dormant for the whole of the child's life, or there may be just one outbreak of blisters, or it could turn into a recurring problem. Certain conditions bring the virus out into the open. An outbreak of blisters is more likely to occur if the child is feeling nervous, if they are unwell, run down, malnourished, if the weather is hot, or if they have another viral infection such as flu, chickenpox, measles, and the common cold — hence the term "cold sores."

Signs and Symptoms

- small blisters that come up around the mouth, near the lips, or inside the mouth, on gums, throat, nostrils, or elsewhere on the face
- the blisters eventually rupture, and crust over
- blisters last 7 to 12 days

If you have a child with cold sores there are two main things to remember. Cold sores come up at the same place, and before the blister appears there is a characteristic tingling in the area. If your child can learn to identify this advance signal, treatment can be given right away, and maybe even prevent the cold sore from erupting. At the very least, the outbreak will less severe. Secondly, the cold sores are very contagious — especially the fluid in the blister.

It's very important that when your child has a cold sore, they don't touch it because the infection could then be spread to other parts of their body that they touch afterward. Your child should only use their own washcloth and towel, and avoid kissing.

Cold Sore Mix

This is a mix of neat essential oil. It can be used on children over 2 years of age.

It can be applied to the area when the warning tingle is felt, before the cold sore erupts, or when the cold sore has already appeared. If the sore is open, this will sting, so warn your child before you put it on. Use a fresh cotton swab each time it touches the skin. You will only use a small amount of the following each time.

2 drops camomile german
5 drops geranium
5 drops tea tree

Essential Oils That Help

Melissa	Lavender
Tea tree	Lemon
Geranium	Manuka
Thyme linalol	Camomile german

Other Care

If you use Vaseline or another type of mineral oil as a barrier, you can add eight drops each of manuka, thyme linalol, and camomile german to a 1-ounce tub of Vaseline and mix well.

When to Get Help

Always consult your doctor to get a definite diagnosis. You should get further medical help if the eyes seem to be affected — which is sometimes the case; or if there is a fever; or if the sores become infected with pus and are very red and painful. You should also tell your doctor if your child suffers from repeated cold sore eruptions.

Special note: Encephalitis can be caused by the herpes simplex 1 virus. If your child contracts encephalitis, tell your doctor that your child suffers from cold sores.

Prevention

If you or your child has a cold sore:

- Don't share washcloths, sponges, towels, cups, glasses, or eating utensils.
- Try to prevent your child from touching the cold sore.
- Change pillows or bed linen every day to prevent cross-infection.
- If hot weather makes the cold sore erupt, use double the amount of sunscreen, particularly on the lips.

COLIC

Infantile colic is quite common in babies and in some cases can go on for many months. It's very painful for the baby and distressing for the parents. Babies can be affected whether they're fed from the breast or the bottle. Colic is usually eased when the trapped gas is eventually passed or a bowel movement is made.

Why some babies should get colic, while others do not, is still something of a mystery. There are many theories including: a) what the mother eats, if she's breast-feeding; b) how the baby eats; and c) what measures are taken to "wind" the baby after it has eaten. All may be contributing to the condition. However, even when all these things are done perfectly, babies can still get colic and cry. . . and cry. . . and cry!

Colic is not the only reason babies cry. Check first that your baby is not hungry or in need of a diaper change. Although there seems to be an expectation that "all babies cry," there might be a serious underlying problem that needs medical attention.

Signs and Symptoms

- intense crying, that can go on for hours, usually in the late afternoon or early evening
- the abdomen feels hard to the touch
- the face is flushed; the lips might become pale
- baby may draw legs up to stomach; may clench fists

If winding doesn't work, mothers often intuitively massage over the baby's abdomen to help release the trapped gas. This is best done gently, in small circular movements, 5 to 10 minutes after feeding or winding. It can be done while the baby is clothed.

Essential oils can be used in a massage oil for the baby. Lay the baby down on your knees and remove any restrictive clothing, including the diaper. Using no more than a quarter of a teaspoon of the following mixture at a time, gently massage the abdomen in small, clockwise, circular movements, then turn the baby over and massage the center of the back, again in small, clockwise circles. The baby may be uncomfortable with the massage on the abdomen, but do persist. When massaging the back, you could place the baby on a warm towel. Make sure the towel is not hot. If the legs are drawn up, you could try massaging the legs and the feet.

Massage Oil	Baths	Dill Herb Water
First mix the essential oils using these proportions: 5 drops coriander 3 drops cardamom 2 drops dill Bottle the essential oils for future use. When required, mix one drop only in $^1/_2$ a teaspoon almond oil — and use half this amount per application.	To help relax the spasm, add $^1/_4$ of a teaspoon the following mix to a warm bath: 1 teaspoon almond oil 1 drop lavender 1 drop cardamom Put the $^1/_4$ teaspoon in the bath. It will float on the surface. Scoop it into your hand and rub over the baby's tummy while in the bath. Make sure none splashes into the baby's eyes or on their face.	Add 1 teaspoon of the following mixture to 4 ounces slightly warm, boiled water in a bottle, for baby to drink. Put in a small bowl: 1 handful fresh dill herb 1 handful fresh mint herb $^1/_4$ teaspoon fennel seeds Pour $^1/_2$ pint boiling water over these, then add 1 teaspoon honey, mix a little, cover with a plate and leave to cool. Strain and bottle. As directed above: use only 1 teaspoon in 4 ounces of water.

Essential Oils That Help

Cardamon   Dill
Coriander

When to Get Help

In most babies the colic will ease after around 4 months of age. If not, help should be sought. If the baby has unusual bowel movements it might mean there are intestinal problems and a doctor should be consulted. If the baby vomits up his or her food on a regular basis, help should be sought, but if the vomiting is projectile — it comes out of the mouth with force and goes some distance — this can indicate a serious problem and medical attention should be sought immediately.

Prevention

- If breast feeding, the mother can try reducing her intake of caffeine and/or gaseous sodas, dairy products, onions, garlic, cabbage, and spicy foods.
- After feeding and winding, put 1 drop of dill essential oil on a tissue and tuck it under the baby's mattress, at the end away from baby's head.

COMPUTER-RELATED PROBLEMS

Computers have not been around long enough for physiologists and psychologists to fully evaluate their effect on our children as they enter adulthood and, eventually, their senior years. Many children today are becoming obsessed with the computer and spend far too long on it. Some parents tell me their children won't eat unless food is taken to them while they sit chatting on E-mail or playing games. Some children are spending all their free time at the computer, as well as using them at school. This can lead to various problems, especially if the child is accessing information their parents would disapprove of.

Parents are perhaps most worried about the type of information available on the internet — especially of a sexual or violent nature. But the computer can be the source of other, more physical concerns, such as radiation in terms of electrical and magnetic emissions — including ELF (extremely low emissions), and VLF (magnetic fields, electrical fields, static electricity fields). Studies have shown that these magnetic fields do have biological effects, particularly on the growth of various cells and tissue, hormones, brain chemicals, and functioning.

Working at a computer for long periods also causes obvious physical problems such as repetitive strain from working on the keyboard with the fingers and hands, visual disturbance caused by the glare of the screen, tinitus and other hearing problems caused by the continual low buzz of the hard disk drive, and asthma exacerbated by an increased number of dust particles in the dry atmosphere.

The two following lists outline the psychological and physical problems that may affect children who spend too long on the computer.

Signs and Symptoms — Emotional

- noncommunicative; irritability; abusiveness; distancing themselves from family; "nobody understands me" syndrome; sadness; having no feelings; emotional outbursts for no apparent reason; hopelessness; insomnia; becoming secretive; getting up to chat on-line when the family has gone to bed

Signs and Symptoms — Stress

- irritability; grinding teeth; muscle tension; fatigue — but unable to sleep; changes in appetite; aggression; shallow breathing

---

Room Diffuser Spray

Use essential oils in the room methods when your child is at the computer. If using the spray method, make sure none of the water droplets fall onto the computer or keyboard.

The best to use at this time are those extracted from leaves and trees, and oxygenate the atmosphere, such as:

Petitgrain, cypress, pine, fir

Also consider using the following:

Eucalyptus — to help with the radiation and assist in breathing
Lavender — to help insomniacs
Lemon — to help focus and concentration while completing school projects and homework

---

Other Care

Limit the length of time younger children spend on the computer. Make sure your child's computer has a glare control screen. Ensure no reflected light is appearing on the screen, and reorganize room lighting so your child is not having to strain their eyes. They should sit on a well-designed ergonomic chair, with a backrest, and work with their elbows on the desk, supporting the wrists. Most emissions come out of the back of the computer, so make sure the back is against an external wall and not a seating or sleeping area. Radiation increases in dry, hot places, so make sure the air is humid, and put plants in the room such as the peace lily and spider plant — both are easily available, they are often found in supermarkets.

Increase your child's intake of vitamins C and E, as ELF emissions are thought to increase the incidence of free radicals in the body. Give your child lots to drink while they're working on the computer, making sure no cups or cans are put on the computer desk where they can be knocked over onto the keyboard.

Prevention

There was a time when we could see who our child was talking to, and take steps to prevent that association if we disapproved. With the Internet and

E-mail, those days have gone. Even the children themselves don't know who they're "talking" to, and pedophiles may be masquerading as children in "chatrooms." In truth, we don't know who is at the end of the line or what thoughts they are putting into our child's head. Moreover, the Internet is full of all kinds of information — some educational and some very dangerous. Have we any idea what our child is learning through the Internet? Spend time with your child on the computer, asking what they have found on the Internet. If you can talk about it with them, it may prevent a "them and us" situation — "they", the parents don't know what's going on, while "us" kids do.

We must also ask ourselves, as parents, do we encourage our child to use the computer because we feel secure knowing where they are, and where they are not — on the street, getting into gangs, meeting the wrong people, drinking, or taking drugs. Are we encouraging our children to make friends on the computer instead of encouraging them to interact with positive real-life human beings?

CONSTIPATION

Although constipation is usually thought of as the absence of stools for a time, it's more accurately defined as stools with a hard texture. It can be caused by a change in dietary habits, stress, or earlier toilet training. The stools become hard and pebble-like. Babies often have constipation when eating solids for the first time. If the child has a fever the stools may be harder than normal because the body absorbs fluid from wherever it can to compensate for the lack of water in the body.

Signs and Symptoms

- dry, hard stools: pebble-like
- stools difficult to pass

Tummy Rub

First, feel around your child's lower abdomen to see if there is any tenderness in the area. If there is, see your physician right away. If all is well, prepare the following mix:

1 teaspoon vegetable oil
2 drops mandarin
2 drops lemon
1 drop petitgrain

Use a small amount each time. Massage the whole of your child's abdomen in gentle movements, working around the umbilicus in a clockwise direction.

Essential Oils That Help

Mandarin   Petitgrain
Lemon   Grapefruit

Other Care

Give your child plenty of plain water to drink, sweetened with a little honey, if they prefer. Let your child's body pass the stools in it's own time; don't tell your child they have to go to the bathroom at a certain time of day. Teach your child to take their time on the toilet or potty. To prevent them from getting bored, read them a story, have them read to you, or listen to music together — do anything to encourage them to stay put, particularly if they are very active children.

When to Get Help

As suggested earlier, check your child's lower abdomen to see if there is any tenderness in the area. If there is, see your physician right away. Also get medical help if there's any blood in the stools; or stomach pains; or if the constipation lasts for longer than a few days.

Prevention

- Give your child plenty of water to drink.
- Give your child lots of fiber, such as prunes, fruit, cereal, bran, bananas, corn, and wholemeal bread.

COUGH

See also: Allergies, Asthma, Bronchitis, Croup, Tonsillitis, Whooping Cough

Coughing is not a condition as such, it's a symptom of some other problem within the body. The coughing reflex is the body trying to clear irritating material from the throat or airways, and is proof that the body's defense system is working as it should. We all cough sometimes, but when coughing is excessive, we know something is wrong.

Signs and Symptoms

- the sound, depth, and source of the cough can indicate where the body's defense system is working, and where the cause of the trouble is located
- the cough may come from the chest or from the throat
- the cough sounds like gurgling as mucus is removed from the air ways

Cough Mix
There are several ways in which the cough mix can be used. Mix the following oils, using these proportions and bottle: 10 drops ravensara 5 drops niaouli 10 drops eucalyptus radiata

Chest and Back Rub	Steam Bowl	Tissue, Pillow, or P.J.s
Rub over the chest and back. Dilute the chest mix of essential oils above in vegetable oil, using the following amounts, depending on the age of the child. Only use a small amount of your diluted oil each time you apply: under 2 years old 4 drops in 1 tablespoon vegetable oil 3–7 years 6 drops in 1 tablespoon vegetable oil 8–11 years 8 drops in 1 tablespoon vegetable oil This can be used at any time, but before bed is the most effective. The rub may help the body loosen any mucus, so the coughing may temporarily get worse as the body rids itself of the mucus as part of the healing process.	To help the child breathe easily during the night, put 8 drops of the essential oils cough mix onto a bowl of steaming hot water and leave in the child's room as they go to sleep. Place out of reach of children and keep pets away.	To help the child breathe easily during the night, put one drop of the cough mix of essential oils on: • a tissue and tuck under the pillow (or) • on the pillow, away from the eye area (or) • on the chest area of the pajamas

Essential Oils That Help

Eucalyptus radiata
Niaouli
Ravensara
Thyme linalol
Camomile german

Essential Oils That Help Aid Sleep

Lavender
Neroli
Ormenis Flower (Camomile maroc)

Other Care

Keep your child warm, and give them plenty to drink. They should avoid doing highly active games or sports, and stay away from areas where people are smoking cigarettes. Moist air can be very helpful. Use a humidifier or, if you don't have one, put a small bowl of steaming hot water in the child's room, out of reach of children or pets, or alternatively put a wet towel or other cloth over a hot radiator.

When to Get Help

All children under one year of age who have a cough should be examined by a physician. If the child is over one year of age, get medical advice if the coughing lasts for more than 24 hours; or if there is a temperature; or fever; or the child has difficulty in breathing in or out. If a cough lasts over one week, it is imperative the child is seen by a doctor.

CRADLE CAP (SEBORRHEA DERMATITIS)

Cradle cap is a skin irritation that affects babies. It's caused by overactivity of the sebaceous glands and dead skin, creating a buildup of a greasy crust on the scalp. It gets worse with perspiration, so keep the baby's head dry and cool, and open to the air whenever possible.

Do not try to remove the crust with your fingers, or rub the scalp vigorously. Instead, brush the hair with a very soft baby's brush. Whatever method you use to treat the condition, it could take up to two weeks to clear completely. Only give treatment while the condition exists.

Signs and Symptoms

- can occur on the head, in the eyebrows, and even behind the ears
- dry, scaly patches becoming flaky
- soft, crusty, yellow scales; can become hard and thick

Plain Oil Method	Aromatherapy Method	Tea Wash
Only use a small amount each time. Gently smooth one of the following over the scalp to help loosen scales. Try to use cold-pressed organic oils. almond oil or sunflower oil	Only use a small amount each time. Gently smooth over the scalp to help loosen scales. Mix together: $1/2$ ounce avocado oil $1/2$ ounce jojoba oil 1 drop tea tree 1 drop orange 1 drop lemon Leave for a few minutes then shampoo off with a mild shampoo. Be careful not to get the oil or shampoo in baby's eyes, or on baby's face.	Add 1 teaspoon of the following "tea" to the final rinse water when washing the baby's hair: $1/2$ pint of water juice of half a lemon 1 handful fresh rosemary 1 handful fresh thyme Put the herbs in a bowl with the lemon juice. Boil the water and pour over the herbs. Leave to cool, then bottle.

Essential Oils That Help

Tea tree   Geranium

Lemon   Orange

When to Get Help

A scaly scalp can also be caused by eczema, psoriasis, or ringworm. If you suspect any of these, consult your doctor. Also, consult your doctor if the scales last longer than 2 to 3 weeks, if they become reddened, or if there are scaly patches in places other than the head, eyebrows, or behind the ears.

CROUP

See also: Allergies, Colds, Cough, Laryngitis

The main symptom of croup is a strange sounding cough, rather like a seal barking — a kind of croaking. The most likely cause is an infection of the airways, but a croaking sound can also be made if the child has swallowed an object that has become stuck in their throat.

Croup is an infection that is usually caused by a virus, which makes the upper part of the airways swollen. When air passes through the airways it causes the strange sound and cough. Croup can follow after an infection like bronchitis. It mostly affects children between the ages of 6 months and 3 years.

Signs and Symptoms

- often starts during the night, when it can seem worse
- difficulty in breathing; chest seems to be deflating more than usual
- when the child inhales, there's a high-pitched wheezing noise (stridor)
- often accompanied with sore throat, hoarse voice, and/or fever
- the child may gag, or vomit
- the child is irritable and tired

Croup Mix
First mix these essential oils together: 15 drops niaouli 15 drops ravensara 10 drops thyme linalol 10 drops palmarosa The mix can be used in the two methods below.

Chest and Back Massage	Pillow or P.J.'s
Dilute 10 drops of the croup mix of essential oils in 1 tablespoon of vegetable oil. Only use a small amount of this each time to massage over the chest and back.	Put one drop of the croup mix of essential oils on the pillow, away from the eye area or on the chest area of the pajamas

---

Steamy Room

The only practical way to get a room full of steam is to run a very hot bath with the door tightly shut. Put a chair in the bathroom, where you can sit with the child on your knee. This is a good time to read a book with them — do not leave the child alone. Add the following essential oils to the hot bath water.

10 drops niaouli
10 drops eucalyptus radiata

Warning: *This bath is not intended to bathe in. The aim is to create an essential oil steamy atmosphere for your child to inhale.*

Essential Oils That Help

Eucalyptus radiata
Niaouli
Ravensara
Thyme linalol
Camomile german
Palmarosa

Essential Oils That Help Aid Sleep

Lavender
Neroli
Marjoram
Camomile maroc

Other Care

Cool moist evening air appears to help during attacks, make sure the child is appropriately dressed and kept warm. At night, add more pillows so your child is propped up in bed. It is important that you stay calm during a coughing attack — it's hard enough for the child, and it doesn't help if they see you are panicked!

When to Get Help

If you think your child's cough could be a result of them having swallowed something call emergency services right away.

Consult your doctor if your child has a temperature, their face has a grayish color, they cannot breathe, they refuse to drink liquids, or if their cough continues more than three days. It may be necessary for the child to be given oxygen.

Prevention

- If your child has bronchitis, shows sign of a respiratory infection, or a croup-like cough, keep them home from school, and make all efforts to deal with the infection.

CUTS AND GRAZES (MINOR)

Children are forever getting themselves into minor accidents as they run around, indoors and out — and cuts and grazes are often the result. Some cuts bleed quite a lot and until the bleeding stops you won't really know the extent of the damage. A deep cut will need to be sutured — stitched up by a professional — and ideally this should be done within 8 hours. Most usually though, children suffer minor cuts and grazes that can be treated at home.

If there's a lot of bleeding, apply pressure to the area with a clean absorbent piece of material to help stop the flow. If the cut is on a limb, hold the injured part up for a while to lessen blood flow to the area.

Signs and Symptoms

- cuts: there's a break in the skin, usually with some bleeding
- cuts: a puncture of the skin caused by the removal of a splinter or other object
- grazes: the top layer of skin has been removed by scraping on a hard surface — may ooze a clear fluid, or bleed slightly in spots

Cuts and Grazes Mix

You can pretty much guarantee that if there's a child in the home you'll need some cuts and grazes mix.

Bottle these simple ingredients for when the need arises:

50 drops lavender
50 drops tea tree

This mix can be kept for up to two years if stored properly and left undiluted.

Washing

With all cuts and grazes, it's extremely important to remove all traces of dirt or grit and the only way this can be done is by washing the area thoroughly. The child may not like it, but it has to be done. Use warm water, and if there's dirt inside the cut, flush it out using any super clean utensil that suits the job.

Add 10 drops of the cuts and grazes mix to the water you use to wash the area. It is an antiseptic and will also help to calm down the child.

Gauze Dressing	Band-Aid Dressing
Put 3 drops of the cuts and grazes mix on a gauze dressing. Alternatively, use lavender on it's own. Place the dressing directly over the cut or graze, and bandage.	Put 1 drop of the cuts and grazes mix (or 1 drop of lavender) onto the dressing part of the Band-Aid that will cover the wounded area.
Expose the cut or graze to the air as much as possible and apply the gauze dressing twice a day.	Don't put the essential oils directly on the cut itself as this will sting and it is unnecessary.

Aftercare
Change the dressing often and leave the wound exposed to the air as much as possible. If the grazed area is very large use the gauze dressing method.
To help with the healing process and keep infection at bay, smear 1 drop of the cuts and grazes mix (or 1 drop lavender) in a circle surrounding the cut or graze. Apply it on unbroken skin around the area, not directly on the cut or graze. If there is swelling, wrap a few ice cubes in a towel and gently hold it against the affected area.

Essential Oils That Help

Lavender   Pine
Tea Tree   Lemon
Manuka   Eucalyptus radiata
Niaouli

When to Get Help

Go for medical help right way if the wound seems to be more than half an inch deep into the tissue; if the cut is jagged and cannot be cleaned properly; or if the bleeding does not stop after 10 minutes of applying pressure with a clean cloth or dressing.

Get medical help if the wound does not heal or if an infection develops and there is pus, swelling, or more tenderness and redness in the area than before, and possibly a fever.

If you see any red lines extending outwards from the cut or graze, do not hesitate, and go immediately to your doctor.

Prevention

There's not much you can do to prevent children having cuts and grazes — that's kids for you! What you can do is help prevent the child from getting tetanus by making sure your child has regular immunizations. Check with your doctor that your child's tetanus immunization is current and up to date.

DANDRUFF

See also: Cradle Cap

Children have dandruff for different reasons. It may just be a buildup of cells on the scalp, or it may be a sign of eczema, psoriasis, or a fungal infection. Head lice are a parasitic infestation of the scalp, and the empty egg-shells left by the small creatures can look very much like dandruff. Children of all ages can have dandruff, which sometimes also affects the eyebrows.

Signs and Symptoms

- white flakes of dead skin on the scalp and hair, which fall onto the shoulders
- dead skin can be seen attached to the scalp; if not removed it can build up into crusty areas

Sometimes, when medications and medicated dandruff shampoos are stopped, the symptoms return and can even increase. And so the product must be bought again to keep the symptoms at bay. This is no long-term solution. As an alternative, try the following, natural three part dandruff plan. It needs to be carried out once a week, with no other washes in between. Removing the buildup of dandruff with constant washing only seems to encourage more skin cells to be shed. Instead, leave it alone, and see if the scalp can balance itself out.

The Three Part Dandruff Plan

Part One — The Oil
Mix the following to make an oil to use at night: 1 ounce jojoba oil $^{1}/_{4}$ ounce rose hip seed oil   15 drops red carrot seed oil   *Use only a small amount but make sure it covers all the scalp. Rub it in well. This mix may stain your bed linen, so use an old pillow case. In the morning, use the shampoo.*

Part Two — The Shampoo

Shampoo the oil out in the morning. Use the gentlest, most natural, shampoo you can find. There are products for babies, children, and non-perfumed brands for sensitive skin. Ideally, use a shampoo that uses coconut derivatives, or the foaming agent from soap wort, rather than other detergents. Essential oils can be mixed directly in with the shampoo. The following amounts are for 4 ounces of shampoo:

10 drops tea tree
10 drops manuka
5 drops myrtle

Then rinse.

Part Three — The Final Rinse

After shampooing, rinse the hair thoroughly. Then apply this final rinse, leave it in the hair. The following amount would be enough for at least eight final rinses.

8 ounces water
26 drops lemon
5 drops tea tree

Shake well, then pour through an unbleached paper coffee filter, and bottle for future use.

Essential Oils That Help

Myrtle
Tea tree
Manuka
Lemon
Cypress
Carrot seed (red)

Other Oils That Help

Jojoba
Borage
Almond
Rose hip seed

When to Get Help

Get medical advice if the child has eczema or psoriasis anywhere on their body; if there is a fungal skin infection; or if you suspect head lice.

DEHYDRATION

The body is made up of 80 percent water, which helps to move vital nutrients around the body. When the body is starved of water we quickly deteriorate. When a child vomits, has diarrhea, or a fever, precious fluids are being lost and dehydration can result.

The most obvious reason a child becomes dehydrated is that they have not been drinking enough. Pure water is by far the best liquid for children, and they do like it, if offered. Pure fruit juice is sugar-laden, but it can be diluted with water. Others drinks contain artificial sweeteners; caffeine; and chemicals for color, preservative, and flavor that aren't exactly known for doing the body any good.

Dehydration is serious! Any child with vomiting and diarrhea should be given immediate medical help, both to help rid the body of whatever infection is causing these symptoms, and to get the right levels of fluid back into the body.

Signs and Symptoms

- dry lips and mouth
- vomiting or diarrhea that lasts more than 5 hours
- drowsiness; sleepiness
- the urine may be dark and smelly — when it becomes clearer, that's a good sign

If your child gets dehydrated, for whatever reason, give them frequent sips of water, even if it passes straight through them. If no water is available, give them whatever fluid you have.

If you are taking your child camping or hiking, or for some other reason away from a city with medical facilities, make sure you carry the crucial ingredients of a dehydration fluid, just in case the child gets sick while away. Don't even think about cutting out the sugar or glucose — that's needed to help with the absorption of salt.

Dehydration Drink

Sip one glass at a time.

1 pint water
$1/_2$ teaspoon salt
4 teaspoons glucose powder (or 6 teaspoons sugar)

Stir until dissolved. Add a little fruit juice if the child refuses to drink the dehydration mix on its own.

Other Care

Make your child sip drinks as drinking too quickly may cause your child's stomach to reject the liquid. "Little and often" is the rule for dehydration. Don't allow your child to get overheated.

When to Get Help

As soon as you can.

DIAPER RASH

This is a common condition that can affect all babies, especially those with sensitive skin, prone to allergies, infantile eczema, or psoriasis. A baby might also be allergic to certain chemical baby wipes, cleaning materials, detergents, and soaps. Babies who have candida (sometimes induced by antibiotics) can also develop a rash.

Diaper rash is most commonly caused by wearing wet or soiled diapers for long periods of time. Feces can break down the urine components and release ammonia into the area. If not treated, diaper rash can become severe and infected with bacteria or fungi. If this happens, the rash will have small, blister-like raised areas or small, pus-infected spots. Action must be taken immediately to stop the spread of infection.

At all times, avoid putting harsh, dry material in contact with the area because they cause more discomfort.

Signs and Symptoms
- affects buttocks, creases of the leg, groin area, and genitals
- redness of skin, inflammation, rashes of various types, scaly patches, or rough skin

Prior to Treatment
Rinse off urine and/or feces as soon as possible with mild soap and water. Use cotton wool, making sure nothing is left on the skin. Pat the area dry using a clean, soft natural material, such as muslin or cheesecloth.

After Washing	*Diaper Rash Oil*	*Baths*
Add to the final rinse water a true herbal hydrolat of camomile roman or lavender. *If not available, make your own water. Follow the directions on page 12, using:* *4 drops camomile german* *4 drops lavender* *in one pint water*	*Heat 3 ounces organic jojoba oil and 1 ounce organic olive oil. Leave to get cold. While cooling, mix:* *8 drops camomile german* *4 drops lavender* *4 drops of ravensara* *(If candida is the cause, add 8 drops tea tree to the mix.)* *Now mix the essential oils into the cold vegetable oils. Apply a small amount at each diaper change until the rash heals completely. Try to avoid the penis and testicles or vulva area. Do not use over cuts or cracks in the skin.*	*Mix together:* *1 drop camomile german* *1 drop lavender* *1 tablespoon full-fat milk* *Then add to the surface of the bath water and swish around well. During the bath avoid getting the oil on baby's face and eyes.*

Essential Oils That Help

In General:
Camomile german
Camomile roman
Lavender
Palmarosa
Yarrow

With Infected Pustules:
Lavender
Ravensara
Thyme linalol
Tea tree

With Candida Albicans:
Geranium
Manuka
Tea tree
Thyme linalol

Other Care

In General:

1 or 2 drops camomile german can be added to each tablespoon of zinc oxide cream.

With Infected Pustules (spots):

Colloidal silver solution (see page 13) can be combined with essential oils.

With Candida Albicans:

Natural (non flavored), bioactive yogurt can be combined with tea tree and manuka essential oils and applied over the affected area of skin.

When to Get Help

If pus can be seen in small spots, or there are blister-like areas, see a doctor before treating with anything, or if the condition does not improve within four days.

Prevention

- Combine 4 ounces of organic almond oil and 1 ounce of organic olive oil, and gently apply a tiny amount after each diaper change. Or apply another water-repellent oil or cream.
- It is important to get air to the area at least once a day. Leave the diaper off for a time, when it's practical.
- Change diapers frequently.
- Keep the skin dry (apart from oils or creams as mentioned above).

DIARRHEA

See also: Dehydration

Diarrhea is the name given to runny, loose stools. It could be caused by many things, including bacterial and viral stomach infections, stress, or an allergic reaction to a food or medication. Diarrhea is a possible symptom of many conditions including colds, flu, ear infection, and sore throats. If it continues for a long time, your child may become dehydrated.

Young babies, particularly if breast-fed, may have soft stools — this is normal. If your child has no symptoms other than diarrhea, don't worry as it will probably pass. If your child is continually passing loose stools, even after a drink of water, seek help as this is not normal.

Signs and Symptoms

- variously colored runny stools
- fluid being passed anally

Tummy Rubs		
Use a small amount to rub over the whole of your child's abdominal area. Choose the appropriate mix.		
Viral Infection	**Food Poisoning**	**Stress**
Dilute the following essential oils in 1 tablespoon vegetable oil:	*Dilute the following essential oils in 1 tablespoon vegetable oil:*	*Dilute the following essential oils in 1 tablespoon vegetable oil:*
3 drops thyme linalol *2 drops lavender* *1 drop tea tree*	*2 drops camomile german* *3 drops peppermint* *1 drop eucalyptus radiata*	*1 drop camomile roman* *2 drops eucalyptus radiata* *3 drops lavender*
Use a small amount each time.	*Use a small amount each time.*	*Use a small amount each time.*

To Calm and Sleep Back Rub

The following mix will help your child sleep if they are distressed:

1 teaspoon vegetable oil
1 drop lavender
1 drop petitgrain

Use $^1/_2$ this amount if your child is under 3 years of age.
Apply on your child's back and gently rub in.

Essential Oils That Help

If it's caused by:

Viral Infection	Food Poisoning	Stress
Tea tree	Thyme linalol	Lavender
Lemon	Tea Tree	Geranium
Lavender	Eucalyptus radiata	Lemon
Eucalyptus radiata	Camomile german	Camomile roman
Thyme linalol	Peppermint	Lavender

Other Care

Let the diarrhea take its course — it may be the body getting rid of a virus or bacteria. To help rehydrate your child's body, give them small sips of an electrolyte solution, available from drug stores or pharmacies. Give your child plenty of water to drink during the day.

When to Get Help

See your physician as soon as possible if there is blood in the stools, stomach pain, vomiting, temperature, or fever. Also get help if the diarrhea lasts longer than 10 hours.

Prevention

- Food poisoning and diarrhea are often caused by poor hygiene. Teach the whole family to wash their hands before touching or preparing foods.

EARACHE AND EAR INFECTION

Earaches and infections are very common during childhood and can be extremely painful. They can affect children of all ages and are as common as colds in those under 5 years of age. The events leading up to the pain are important when trying to identify the cause, as this will help decide what treatment is appropriate. An infection may lead to an earache, but you need to question: was it caused by a cold, tonsillitis, or mumps, or by having water in the ear that became infected? Other causes of earache are toothache and sinus problems. Sinus problems can include sinusitis or hay fever. Having a boil or spot in the area can cause earache, as can being out in the cold, wind, or snow. So, it's important to narrow down the reason for the earache, and tell this to your doctor and treat accordingly.

If your child has recurring earaches for no apparent reason, it's likely they have an infection that is not responding to treatment. All earaches should be treated as a potential long-term problem because if they're left untreated, hearing in later life might be impaired. If the pain is persistent, it could indicate an infection or perforated ear drum.

Signs and Symptoms
- pain
- discharge or fluid coming out of ear indicates an infection
- fever, colds and sniffles, irritability, balance problems
- in very young children: pulling or rubbing the ears, crying, distress
- in older children: dizziness

Ear Massage

Massage around the back of the affected ear — outside the ear, on the side of the head — with one of the following mixes:

Earache Mix	Ear Infection Mix No. 1
Use only a small amount each time. $^{1}/_{2}$ *ounce vegetable oil* *10 drops lavender* *5 drops camomile german* *6 drops palmarosa* *3 drops cardamom*	*Use only a small amount each time. If this is not effective, try the stronger ear infection mix No. 2.* $^{1}/_{2}$ *ounce vegetable oil* *3 drops thyme linalol* *3 drops lavender*
Ear Infection Compress	**Ear Infection Mix No. 2**
A warm compress may help with the pain. Put 3 drops thyme linalol and 3 drops lavender on a warm compress, and hold against the ear.	*First mix up these essential oils:* *5 drops thyme linalol* *3 drops lavender* *10 drops camomile roman* *3 drops palmarosa* *Use 3 drops of this mix, diluted in 1 teaspoon vegetable oil. Use only $^{1}/_{2}$ teaspoon per application.*

Essential Oils That Help

Niaouli	Marjoram
Juniper berry	Tea tree
Thyme linalol	Lavender
Camomile roman	

Other Care

Warmth sometimes helps to soothe an earache. Apply warmth to the area by, for example, holding a covered hotwater bottle against the ear, or putting a low temperature heating pad in the child's pillow case. Don't use these methods if boils or spots are present.

When to Get Help

The causes of earache have the potential to be harmful to the child's health, and it's important to get a proper diagnosis. Always get medical advice if there is any loss of hearing, discharge from the ear, a temperature, fever, loss of balance, if the child has a red and sore throat, spots and boils, or if the pain has continued for more than 24 hours.

ECZEMA (ATOPIC DERMATITIS)

Eczema is an itchy skin condition that is often caused by an allergy to certain foods or environmental considerations. It often starts to develop at the time solid foods are introduced into the diet, at around 4 or 5 months of age. If it occurs before then, the child may be allergic to powdered milk, or to breast milk, particularly if it contains allergy producing elements. Most children with infantile eczema grow out of it by the age of 3, however, for some unlucky children they can continue to suffer with eczema into adulthood.

Eczema is closely associated with asthma and hay fever, and the child may have these conditions as well. There is also the genetic factor — if either parent, or grandparents, have these conditions, it may be experienced in the child as eczema.

If the eczema is allergy-based, the most likely sources of the trouble are wheat, dairy products, eggs, pet hair, wool, water softening agents, and clothes softening products. Eczema can also be triggered by stress and anxiety.

Signs and Symptoms
- dry, flaky skin, cracking of the skin, scaly skin
- itching skin, redness
- red rash mainly affecting face, armpits, knees, elbows, hands, and genital area

Soothing Baths

Scratching makes the itch worse, and can cause infection. One of the best ways to reduce the irritation is to have soothing baths. There are several types of baths to choose from.

Vegetable Oil Bath	Anxiety Relieving Bath	Oat Bag Bath
Add 1 tablespoon plain vegetable oil to a bath. It will float on the surface, and moisten the child's skin when they come out of the bath. Be careful not to use anything with wheat germ in it or any other oil produced from a grain. Use one of the following: almond oil jojoba oil grapeseed oil sunflower seed oil	To the vegetable oil used in the Vegetable Oil Bath method, add 2–3 drops of either: lavender or geranium	Put a small amount of organic oats on a square of muslin material. Drop onto the oats: $1/2$ teaspoon jojoba oil 1 drop lavender Tie the bag securely, and place in the bath.

Soothing Lotions

Oil Mix

Use a small amount of the following oil mix on the affected areas of skin, as needed. First mix the following essential oils together:

10 drops lavender
10 drops camomile german
6 drops palmarosa
2 drops bergamot

Then, mix the following vegetable oils together:

2 ounces almond oil
$1/4$ ounce jojoba oil
$1/2$ ounce sunflower seed oil
$1/4$ ounce camellia oil
6 drops evening primrose oil

Now combine the essential oil mix and the vegetable oil mix.

Calamine Lotion Mix

To each 4 ounces calamine lotion, add 2 drops of your chosen essential oil. See the list below.

Essential Oils That Help

Camomile german   Elemi

Yarrow   Ho-wood

Lavender   Palmarosa

Other Care

Use calamine lotion, with or without essential oils. Avoid astringent lotions and mineral-based baby oils.

When to Get Help

As soon as the first sign of eczema appears, make a note of everything new your child has been exposed to, as they may be allergic to some element in its manufacture. Ask yourself whether new food or drinks have been consumed, or a new piece of clothing worn. Also, note whether you have used a new laundry detergent or household cleaner. If an allergy is involved, it could be caused by something obscure, like a new feather or foam pillow. Think of everything new that you can, take it out of the child's environment, and see if things improve.

EPILEPSY (SEIZURES)

The seizures of epilepsy can affect children to varying degrees. Petite mal seizures are the less dramatic kind, with slight shaking and/or the child going into a trance-like state for a time. Grande mal seizures overtake the whole body, and the child may thrash about uncontrollably for several minutes.

Signs and Symptoms
- uncontrolled body movements, over a period of minutes
- slight shaking; far-away look

Brain wave imaging systems have proved that essential oils do have an affect on seizures. At the Queen Elizabeth Hospital in Birmingham, England, Dr. Tim Betts and his team have had great success in reducing patient's epilepsy seizures using the essential oils of jasmine, ylang ylang, camomile, and lavender. The other oils on the list that follows would work equally well.

Whether carried out professionally, or at home by parents and caretakers, aromatherapy treatment should be calming and consistent. Dr. Betts' work has shown that after a period of time and use of a particular essential oil or blend, patients who suffer from seizures may simply be able to sniff from a bottle of the same essential oil or blend used in treatment, to prevent seizures from happening while they are out and about enjoying life.

Massage Oil

Use the following volumes to make the massage oil:

1 ounce vegetable oil
5 drops essential oil

Do not be tempted to use more essential oil than this. It's unnecessary, and it is better to use small amounts with this condition.

Only use a little of the oil at a time and massage the child's back before bed. Use upward stroking movements, towards the neck. Do this twice a week to start with, gradually reducing the number of massages.

While massaging your child, play a tape of gentle music, or relaxing sounds such as woodland bird song or a stream of water.

If the oil you have chosen is having a positive effect in reducing the incidence of seizures, give your child a tissue with a drop of that same essential oil, for them to sniff whenever they feel a seizure might be coming on, or feel anxious.

Essential Oils That Help

Jasmine	Petitgrain
Neroli	Camomile roman
Rose	Geranium

Other Care

Do not move the child unless they are in danger. Do not try to force their mouth open. Loosen any tight clothing. Protect the head. Try to protect the child from injury during the seizure. Place in the recover position when the seizure is over and provide comfort until fully recovered from the seizure.

When to Get Help

Get medical help immediately if the child is having their first seizure or if the child remains unconscious for more than a few minutes. If the child has repeated seizures call emergency services.

FEVER

Fever is a symptom rather than an illness. There are many things a fever could be symptomatic of. In babies, it could be because a tooth is coming through. A fever might result from the flu, a cold, cough, tonsillitis, chicken pox, measles, mumps, food poisoning, or an earache — anything that's been caused by a virus or bacteria. It's the body trying to fight off an infection, a natural process that is, nonetheless, very distressing for children and parents alike.

Signs and Symptoms

- temperature is over 37° Celsius or over 99.5° Fahrenheit, when measured orally (normal temperature for children is 96.8°–98.6°F)
- body feels hot: skin can be hot and sweaty or hot and dry
- red, flushed face, hot hands and feet
- child feels chilly and shivers, although says they feel very hot
- child has no energy, just wants to lie down

Children's temperatures can raise from doing continuous exercise or other strenuous activity, so when taking the temperature for the first time, bear that in mind. Check the temperature every half an hour. Let the child lie down somewhere you can see them and check up on them regularly. Cover them up, but only with a light blanket or sheet. If a child shivers, it's the body using another tool at its disposal to lose heat.

Sponge Method

Prepare a bowl of luke-warm — not cold — water, to which you've added a total of 2 drops essential oil, choosing from the Essential Oils That Help list below. 1 drop lavender and 1 drop eucalyptus radiata are a good mix. Use the water to sponge your child down.

The Vinegar Method for Fevers

The old fashioned European way of dealing with fevers was vinegar, water, and brown paper. Using cloth as an alternative to the brown paper we can update and improve the whole process with essential oil. Prepare with the following:

a bowl of luke-warm water
2 tablespoons vinegar
3 drops lavender

Put a piece of cloth or plain, unprinted brown paper in the bowl, squeeze out, then place it over the forehead of the child, making sure nothing drips into the eyes. When it heats up, remove it, and repeat the procedure.

Compress and Massage

The following method may help your child sleep. Add the following essential oils to a bowl of cool, but not cold, water:

1 drop camomile roman
1 drop lavender
1 drop lemon
1 drop coriander

Dip a compress in the water and squeeze out. Place over your child's back for about 5 minutes. Make sure the water isn't cold, but pleasantly cool to the child. Then dry the skin and massage the back with this oil:

1 teaspoon vegetable oil
2 drops rose otto
1 drop lavender

Essential Oils That Help

Lavender	Eucalyptus radiata
Tea tree	Camomile roman
Lemon	Spearmint

Other Care

Try to make your child as comfortable as possible. Make sure they are not wearing too many clothes. A luke-warm bath is cooling, if the child wants to take it, but never force them to have a bath if they're not feeling well. If necessary, sponge them down on the bed instead. Never use cold water as this may force the body to work harder and actually raise the temperature. Give your child lots of fluids to drink, including fruit juice to sip. Watch for signs of dehydration (see Dehydration).

When to Get Help

Get medical help if the temperature reaches 103 degrees, or has been high for longer than 10 hours, if there are other symptoms present, or if the child has a convulsion, or if it is under 3 months of age.

FIFTH DISEASE (ERYTHEMA INFECTIOSUM)

Fifth disease is a contagious rash caused by a virus — Human Parovirus B19. The rash generally lasts no longer than 24 days, although in some children it will fade and then reappear. The virus is not harmful to most children, but it can have a bad effect on children with a blood disorder, lowered immunity condition, or cancer. Pregnant women, too, should try to avoid it, as it can cause anaemia or miscarriage

Fifth disease is very common among children of elementary school age, especially during the winter and spring months. It's caught simply by breathing in affected air. Because it's very contagious during the two weeks before the rash appears, it's difficult to control. Once a rash appears, the child is no longer contagious, but by then, the virus could have passed half-way through a school. In warmer climates especially, the rash can appear and then disappear, then appear again and so on, for weeks. This can make it difficult to always know if the child is contagious or not.

Things are further complicated by the fact that there are often no obvious symptoms to Fifth disease at all — the child just feels generally not well, with aches and pains and irritability. The child might have a slight fever, and less energy — just wanting to lie around all day. Fifth disease can even be mistaken for the common cold.

Signs and Symptoms
- rash appears on the cheeks
- in some children, the rash may spread to other parts of the body, such as the legs and arms
- older children often have no rash, but instead get aches and pains in their joints

Especially if you have other children in the household, or a pregnant woman, spray the air with antiviral essential oils; see Antiinfectious Air Spray on page 37. Baths can help soothe the skin if your child has the rash, and there are several to choose from. Aside from those below, you could try one of the baths for Chickenpox or Eczema.

Oat Bath	Soothing Bath
Here is an oat bath that can be prepared quickly. Add the following to the bath water and swish around well before the child gets in: 1 large tablespoon oatmeal 1 handful sea salt 1 drop lavender 1 drop camomile german 1 drop tea tree	First, add these essential oils to a cup of bicarbonate of soda: 2 drops lavender 1 drop camomile german 1 drop helichrysum Then mix well with a spoon before adding to the bath water.

Adolescent Joint Rub

If your child is an adolescent with joint pains caused by Fifth disease, mix the following together and rub a little over all the joints just before the child has a warm bath:

2 ounces vegetable oil
5 drops rosemary
7 drops lavender
8 drops marjoram
5 drops thyme linalol

Essential Oils That Help

Lavender	Lemon
Camomile roman	Thyme linalol
camomile german	Helichrysum
Geranium	Cardamom

Other Care

Spray the air with antiviral essential oils. See Antiinfectious Air Spray on page 37.

When to Get Help

Get medical attention if your child also has a blood disorder, or a condition with lowered immunity, or cancer.

Prevention

- If a child in the home has Fifth disease keep them away from other children.
- Spray the air with antiviral essential oils. See Antiinfectious Air Spray on page 37.

FROSTBITE

When the temperature is extremely cold, there's a risk of frostbite. It's caused by ice crystals forming in the fluid and tissues of the body, which stop the flow of blood to the affected areas — usually the fingers, toes, nose, and ears.

Signs and Symptoms

- severe pain in extremities, including fingers, toes, nose, ears
- skin color is first red, then affected area becomes numb
- skin may turn a grayish white-to-yellow, and blister
- if the skin turns black, it is dying, and there is possibility of gangrene setting in

If frostbite occurs, quickly cover the child with as much clothing as possible — especially over the extremities. Do not rub the affected area in an attempt to bring heat into it. Instead, put that area into a bowl of warm — not hot — water, and continue until the skin starts to turn pink. Slowly add hot water to the bowl as needed, to keep the water warm. Essential oils can be added — use ten drops in a bowl of warm water, choosing from the list below.

If it's the nose that's affected, get any piece of cloth and soak it in warm water, squeeze it out, put 1 drop of geranium on it, and place that over the nose while still warm. Keep repeating until the nose has thawed out and returned to its normal color. Noses first go red then gradually loose their color. Still carry out this warm compress method if the nose is red.

Skin Oil

After using the warm water bowl or nose compress method and the skin is the correct color again, gently apply a small amount of the following oil:

1 tablespoon vegetable oil
10 drops geranium
10 drops black pepper

The amount you use will depend upon the areas affected. This amount will cover a very large area. You will probably not need to use it all. Use three times a day.

Essential Oils That Help

Geranium   Marjoram
Black pepper   Ginger
Helichrysum

When to Get Help

Get medical help as soon as possible.

Prevention

- If it's cold, wrap your child up very well with waterproof boots or shoes, two pairs of socks and gloves, ear muffs, a hat, and a thick scarf that can protect the nose.

GROWING PAINS

Children of any age can suffer with growing pains. They may say the pain is "all over," and not in any particular place. Or they may say the pain is "in the bones." Growing pains can be anything from a dull ache to extreme pain. Thankfully, they rarely last a long time. Nobody really knows what causes growing pains, although it's fairly clear that in some cases it's because the bones, ligaments, and muscles are growing at different rates. Growing pains often occur at night, and can even wake a child up.

Signs and Symptoms

- aches in the limbs, source of pain is often uncertain
- muscular soreness
- pain: between the joints, in the shin and other bones, and other areas of the body
- often felt during the night, or after daytime strenuous physical activity

The first thing to do is rub your hands all over the area the child says is aching. Feel for any swelling or lumps under the skin. If you apply slight pressure around any joint near the area of concern, it will help you determine whether there has been any injury or damage. Ask your child questions to find out if anything happened during the day to cause the pain. Did they fall over, for example, or hurt themselves playing sports? If you find no injury, or reason for the pain, proceed with the growing pains home remedies.

Growing pains can be very distressing for children, who have a great imagination and can get worried about pain that seems to have no cause. Reassure your child that everything is going to be okay, and give them lots of comfort. Massage your child's aching limb/s and, if it's nighttime, try to stay with them until they fall asleep. If it's a small child, you may want to put them in your bed.

Massage Oil

Use a small amount of the following oil to gently massage the arms or legs:

1 tablespoon vegetable oil (or calendula infused oil)
3 drops camomile roman
2 drops marjoram

Use only light pressure with upward stroking movements and no pressure at all on the downward strokes.

Apply Warmth

Warmth applied to the aching area may bring some relief. This can be done before massaging the limb, or after, or at any other time. Use warm, dry compresses or towels to wrap around painful limbs. Or use a warm hot water bottle, or a wheat bag, to hold against more specific areas.

Warm Baths

Warm baths can bring relief to aching limbs. If your child comes home from school complaining of growing pains, run them a bath and add the following mix:

1 teaspoon vegetable oil
3 drops lavender
1 drop marjoram

The oil will float on the surface of the water. Show your child how to scoop the oil into the palm of their hand and gently rub it into the painful area of the arm or leg.

A warm bath before bed will help bring a good night's sleep. Refer to the chart on page 15 for the recommended number of drops to use for the different age groups, and choose from the essential oils below.

Essential Oils That Help

Camomile german   Lavender
Camomile roman   Calendula infused oil
Marjoram

When to Get Help

Seek immediate medical help if your child feels pain in the left side of their upper chest. Joint pain and severe arm or leg pain or swelling can be signs of other conditions such as rheumatism and juvenile arthritis. If the pain continues for longer than 24 hours, consult your physician. Also seek medical help if the pain is accompanied by a high temperature or fever.

HAND, FOOT, AND MOUTH DISEASE

Hand, foot, and mouth disease is a viral infection that causes blister-type sores in the mouth, on the hands, and on the feet. It's more likely to occur during the kindergarten years, when children routinely put their fingers in their mouths, although children up to around the age of ten can also get it. Infected children spread the virus by touching the blisters, then toys and other objects, or another child. It can also be spread by the child sneezing and coughing, and not washing their hands after going to the bathroom. Hand, foot, and mouth disease usually lasts around 10 days. It spreads faster in the summer months.

Signs and Symptoms

- fever with temperature up to around 103°F degrees, sore throat, feeling not well, runny nose, cold-type symptoms
- blisters appear in the mouth and form painful sores when they break
- eating is difficult
- a blister-type rash may appear on the hands and feet, and spread to the palms of the hands and soles of the feet
- a blister-type rash may possibly appear on the legs and buttocks

As soon as hand, foot, and mouth disease is suspected, apply one drop of thyme linalol slightly diluted in one drop of vegetable oil over the glands of the neck, then apply a small amount of vegetable oil over the top. Children with sensitive skin may react to this with reddening of the skin but this will pass. If your child is old enough to understand the concept of rinsing their mouth and spitting out — and can actually do it — try the mouthwash that follows. If there is a chance your child might swallow the wash, do not use it.

Hand, Foot, and Mouth Wash

This wash is for the blisters in the mouth, but only if your child is old enough to spit the mixture out. First, mix the following:

1 ounce aloe vera juice
1 ounce honey water (water with 1 teaspoon of honey mixed in)
1 drop cypress
1 drop ravensara

Shake the ingredients together, in a bottle. The essential oils will still float on the surface. Continue to shake vigorously, then pour through an unbleached paper coffee filter into a measuring jug, and rebottle.

Add one teaspoon of the mix to a small 6-ounce glass of water and have your child rinse their mouth, making sure they spit it out afterward. They should not swallow the mouth wash. Repeat as often as possible.

Nighttime Massage Oil

Make the essential oil mix below, use only 3 drops of the mix, diluted in 1 teaspoon vegetable oil. Massage over your child's body, avoiding the genital area, every evening before bedtime.

5 drops thyme linalol
5 drops geranium
5 drops niaouli
5 drops helichrysum

Essential Oils That Help

Thyme linalol
Geranium
Ravensara
Tea tree
Niaouli
Eucalyptus radiata

Lavender
Helichrysum
Cypress
Ormenis flower (Camomile maroc)
Camomile german

Other Care

Have your child eat bland food, excluding anything acidic, such as oranges, tomatoes, and certain soda drinks. Give them lots of cool drinks to help with the soreness. Fluid is very helpful at this time. Make honey popsicles by adding a spoon of honey to melon or other fruit juices and freezing. Be careful your child does not share cups or food utensils with other people.

When to Get Help

As this disease has similar symptoms to other conditions be sure to get a proper medical diagnosis. Get help if the fever goes over 102°F degrees, or if the blisters do not clear up after 14 days.

Prevention

- Try to stop your child sucking their fingers or thumb.
- Teach your child good hygiene.

HAY FEVER

Hay fever is an allergic reaction to pollen, and is at its worse during the spring and early summer. In the autumn, weeds such as ragweed can also provoke an attack. Children who are prone to hay fever often come from families where another member has it, or where there is asthma, eczema, or psoriasis. Hay fever sufferers may also be sensitive or allergic to certain foods or household products.

Signs and Symptoms

- sneezing
- nose congestion
- unable to breathe properly, runny nose, cold-like symptoms
- red, itchy, sore, watering eyes
- stuffy head

Because hay fever affects people in different ways, you'll need to experiment with the essential oils to see which best suit your child. Surprisingly perhaps, the flower essential oils can be very helpful in easing the symptoms, and I've found in my practice that both camomile german and camomile roman work well, as do the other oils on the Essential Oils That Help list below.

Tissue Method

This method can be used with children over 2 years of age. Put one drop of a hay fever mix onto a tissue and give it to your child to inhale during the day. Experiment with both mixes to see which works best for your child.

Mix No. 1	Mix No. 2
Mix together the following. Use one drop only on a tissue:	*Mix together the following. Use one drop only on a tissue:*
4 drops camomile roman 4 drops lemon 2 drops lavender	4 drops geranium 2 drops rosemary 2 drops eucalyptus radiata

Evening Baths	*Diffuser/Burner*
Make up one of the tissue mixes above, and add to the water in evening baths. Use this amount, depending on the age of your child: *Up to 2 years* *1 drop* *2–7 years* *2 drops* *8–11 years* *3 drops* *12 years and over* *4 drops*	*Diffuse these essential oils in your child's bedroom as they go to sleep. Do not leave the diffuser there overnight.* *1 drop helichrysum* *1 drop lavender*

Essential Oils That Help

Lemon   Lavender
Geranium   Neroli
Camomile roman   Tangerine
Eucalyptus radiata   Mandarin
Rosemary   Grapefruit

Other Care

Give your child a small, moist towel or washcloth, secured in a plastic zippered bag, to soothe their eyes during the day. Eye drops may also help. Allergy skin-tests can be arranged for children who suffer from hay fever, and they may help identify the exact causes of your child's attacks.

Prevention

- Keep windows closed when there is a high pollen count.
- Avoid high pollen areas or freshly cut grass.
- Avoid feather-filled pillows and duvets.
- As dust can make the allergy worse, keep the home as dust-free as possible with frequent vacuuming and cleaning.

HEADACHE
See also: Migraine

Most children will complain of headaches now and again, but almost one child in five suffers regularly from headaches although no cause may be found. Headaches can occur because of overtiredness, stress, toothache, tummy ache, earache, colds, and flu. Children may sometimes find it easier to complain of having a headache when there are, in fact, other symptoms they don't want to talk about. Headaches can be symptomatic of more serious disorders, such as high blood pressure, infections, diseases, and head injury.

Any headache where there is also neckache or pain, stiffness, joint pain, fever, vomiting, nausea, or when the child cannot bear bright light, must be treated as an emergency. Get immediate medical help as these may be symptoms of meningitis, encephalitis, or head injury.

Signs and Symptoms
- pain in head — anything from mild ache, to throbbing, pounding, severe pain
- pain described as located in one particular part of head, or all over
- in younger children: irritability, tiredness, crying

Before proceeding, ask your child exactly where the pain is. Go through the list of symptoms in the following section, When to Get Help, asking your child about each in turn. Take their temperature, and ask them if they have a sore throat. Be sure to ask whether they had a fall earlier in the day, or hurt their head in some way. If you are satisfied that your child only has a simple headache then use the following home remedies.

First Steps

Have your child lie down, and make them a warm drink. Then apply to their head a cool compress made using lavender and peppermint water (see page 17).

Headache Mix

Prepare the headache mix using:

10 drops lavender
4 drops camomile roman
10 drops eucalyptus radiata

This mix can be used in diffusers or in oil rubs; use the quantities recommended below.

Diffusers	**Oil Rub**
Use 4 drops of the headache mix above in diffusers.	Dilute 3 drops of the headache mix in 1 teaspoon vegetable oil. Use a small amount, and rub over the neck and upper back. Also smear a tiny amount over both temples, making sure you avoid the eye area.

Essential Oils That Help

Lavender   Camomile
Eucalyptus radiata   Lemon
Petitgrain   Helichrysum
Cardamom   Myrtle
Niaouli

Other Care

Fresh air often helps. The suggested essential oils and treatments can also be used with over the counter children's medications for headaches.

When to Get Help

Get immediate medical help if the headache is accompanied by any of the following: neck ache or pain, stiffness, muscle or joint pain, if the child is sensitive to bright light, had a fever, is vomiting, or has a feeling of nausea. Call your doctor if the headache persists.

HEAD LICE

Head lice have been a nuisance for human beings, especially young ones, since time began. Lice seem to be an inevitable fact of life. Lots of children catch lice at some time, usually in kindergarten or elementary school. It makes no difference whether the hair is spotlessly clean or dirty, or whether it is short and curly or long and straight. Lice will pass from head to head as children sit close to each other in class or as they play. They are also passed from person to person if combs and brushes are shared.

The louse is a six-legged insect, smaller than a match head but visible to the eye. It bites the scalp and feeds on the blood it sucks out. Then it lays eggs in minuscule white shells, about half an inch from the scalp. When the baby louse comes out, the shell stays attached to the hair shaft. These are called *nits*. It's often when finding these shells we become alerted to the fact there are lice in the hair, because unlike dandruff, they cannot be brushed out. The insects themselves are sensitive to light and very good at hiding.

Problems can occur if the child has been scratching their head a lot, and the scalp has become red and irritated, or even infected with bacteria. If the infestation has carried on for a long time, the lymph glands can become enlarged, possibly as an allergic reaction.

Signs and Symptoms
- tiny, white, empty shell-cases, attached to the hair shaft, near the scalp
- very small insects on the scalp and in the hair
- itchy scalp, especially at the nape of the neck and behind the ears

Head lice rarely jump onto infants' hair, possibly because there is not so much of it. But even infants can become affected if other members of the family have lice. Because families are in constant close contact, and may share towels, brushes, and combs, they are often affected at the same time, and the whole family should be treated at the same time.

It's very important to comb the hair with a fine tooth comb. This is the only way to get the lice and nits out of the hair. Some of the head lice combs available on the market only collect the insects themselves, leaving the eggs behind. Flea combs for pets are often better because they're designed for cats, who have very fine hair, and the comb teeth are closer together.

Many of the commercial, chemical preparations should not be used by pregnant women or infants under 3 years of age. The following mix is safe for pregnant women and for infants if the amount used is 50 percent of that used for others. Only treat small babies if they already have head lice. It's unlikely they will catch them if other members of the family are treated. Use 3 drops of the following mixture in your usual baby shampoo and rinse thoroughly.

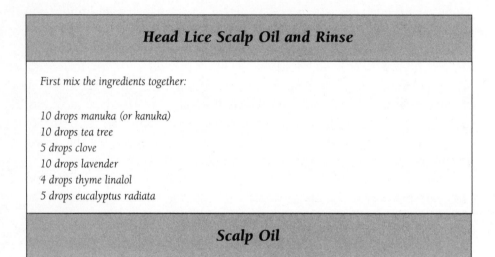

Head Lice Scalp Oil and Rinse

First mix the ingredients together:

10 drops manuka (or kanuka)
10 drops tea tree
5 drops clove
10 drops lavender
4 drops thyme linalol
5 drops eucalyptus radiata

Scalp Oil

Put 10 drops of the head lice scalp oil mix in 1 tablespoon sesame oil and apply it to the scalp. Do not allow the mixture near the eyes, nose, or ears. Cover the hair with a shower cap and leave for half an hour.

Then using a fine tooth comb, gently comb, wiping the comb between each sweep through the hair. Comb the hair in one inch sections. If the hair is long, you'll need to use clips to separate the hair. When you have combed the whole head, wash the hair with a gentle baby shampoo. Then use the following rinse.

Rinse

After shampooing, pour this final rinse through hair, making sure it doesn't get into the eyes, ears, nose, or mouth.

4 ounces water
10 drops head lice mix above

Shake very well before use.

Scalp Calm

If your child's scalp has become irritated because of the biting and possible infection, make up the following:

1 teaspoon jojoba oil
1 drop camomile german
2 drops lavender

Apply directly onto the scalp with your fingertips. Gently separate the hair into sections, so you can reach the whole scalp.

Alternative Method: The Beeswax Barrier

An alternative approach to head lice management is to make a barrier between them and their food source, the scalp. Do not attempt this treatment unless you have the exact ingredients listed below, and follow the directions carefully.

You will need a double boiler. The ingredients are mixed in the top pan of the double boiler. First, melt the beeswax then, while still warm, stir in the castor oil. Keep stirring, while you add the essential oils.

$^1/_4$ ounce natural beeswax (not the white variety)
1 ounce castor oil

While this is still warm, add:

5 drops tea tree
5 drops lavender
5 drops geranium

Mix together well. When cool enough to apply, take a small amount on your fingertips and dab it onto the scalp — not on the hair. If it does get in some hair, and your ordinary shampoo doesn't remove it, try a dandruff shampoo, or a small amount of biodegradable washing liquid.

Essential Oils That Help

Kanuka	Lavender
Manuka	Eucalyptus radiata
Neem	Lemongrass
Rosemary	Thyme linalol
Geranium	

Prevention

There is not much you can do to prevent your child from catching head lice except keeping long hair tied back or in a head band. What you can do is try to prevent it spreading to other members of the family.

- Don't share combs, brushes, towels, pillows, or cushions.
- Without being too obvious about it, try to keep those with head lice away from those without.

HEAT EXHAUSTION

See also: Heat Stroke and Sunburn

When the weather gets very hot children are at risk of heat exhaustion and, in more serious cases, heat stroke. Read the symptoms in that section as well as this, to make sure your child only has heat exhaustion. With heat stroke you need immediate medical attention.

Signs and Symptoms
- dizziness, fainting, fatigue, nausea
- may have raised temperature and perspiration
- thirsty, or may not be thirsty
- irritable, crying

Heat exhaustion is caused by the body overheating due to excessive heat, for example, from being in too much sun, or doing too much exercise while in the sun or an extra warm room. The first thing to do is get the child into a cool, shaded place, preferably indoors. Lay them down, remove most of their clothing, and have them sip water continuously. If you can add a little salt and sugar to the water, dissolving it well, that will help (see Dehydration).

If nothing else is available, put a cool, wet cloth on your child's face, and another on the back of their neck. Refresh the cloths when they heat up. If the child sleeps, that will also help revive them.

Cooling a body down too rapidly is as bad as not cooling it down at all. If you try to cool someone down too quickly they can go into shock. If you use one of the traditional cooling down methods, like compresses or sponging, use cool water — never use ice cold water.

Cooling Comptress Method

Dab a tiny smear of lavender on the back of the child's neck, on the diaphragm solar plexus area (above the belly button), and on both temples, being sure to avoid the eye area.

Put a cool, damp compress or cloth over the back of your child's neck, and cover their body with a light sheet.

Essential Oils That Help

Lavender   Petitgrain
Eucalyptus radiata

When to Get Help

Get medical help if your child's temperature is 101°F or over, or if their body has not cooled down after 30 minutes.

Prevention

In hot weather:

- Make sure your child is always wearing a hat, and their shoulders are covered.
- Keep your child out of the sun as much as possible.
- Make sure your child has plenty to drink. Water is best.

If running or doing sports:

- Make sure your child has periods of rest. If you're out in the sun, bring them into the shade, and cool them down.
- Make sure your child has plenty to drink. Water is best.

HEAT RASH (PRICKLY HEAT)

Heat rash is very common among babies and small children, although anyone at any age can get a heat rash. It happens when the body gets overheated, and over-sweats, causing a blockage in the sweat glands. Babies suffer with it because their sweat glands may not have matured enough to be able to function properly in hot weather.

A heat rash is a collection of tiny blisters that look like tiny pink or red spots. They can come up anywhere on the body, and can be very itchy. Fortunately, home help can often sort out this problem.

Signs and Symptoms

- a red rash anywhere on body, including face, neck, and head
- for babies and infants rash often in folds of skin

As a general rule, try to keep small children's skin dry. On hot days, pat it with a light cotton cloth to absorb sweat. Warm baths are soothing to the skin, but keep the water at just above body temperature — not too cold, as this may cause shock.

Baths
The temperature of the water should be just above body temperature — not cold.

Essential Oil Baths	. . . with Baking Soda
Eucalyptus radiata and lavender are a cooling combination in baths. Make a mix of them, using equal amounts of each. From this, use the following number of drops of the mix, for the different age groups: Up to 2 years 1 drop of the mix 2–7 years 2 drops of the mix 8–10 years 3 drops of the mix 10 years and over 4 drops of the mix	Add just lavender to the baking soda, and mix them together well. Then put them in the bath. Don't put them in separately. Use the following amounts, depending on the age of the child: **Up to 2 years** $1/_4$ cup baking soda and 1 drop lavender **2–7 years** $1/_2$ cup baking soda and 2 drops lavender **8–10 years** $1/_2$ cup of baking soda and 3 drops lavender **10 years and older** 1 cup baking soda and 4 drops lavender

Essential Oils That Help

Lavender   Camomile roman

Eucalyptus radiata

Other Care

Keep an eye on babies in warm weather. Be sure to dress them in loose, cool, clothing. Dress them in cotton — avoid man-made fibers. Open the windows so fresh air can circulate.

When to Get Help

Get help when all home help has failed — and the rash is still there; or if other symptoms develop such as vomiting, head pain, or continual crying.

Prevention

- Keep young babies and infants cool when in the heat, with loose, cotton clothing.
- When possible, let the affected skin be exposed to the air.
- Keep the folds of baby's skin dry.
- Keep bottoms dry.
- Don't use baby products that block baby's pores, avoiding those that are mineral-based.
- Try using corn or rice powders instead of talcum powder, making sure your baby inhales none of the powder.
- The condition of the skin can be made worse by certain ingredients in washing powders and liquids that respond to the heat and sweat, enzymes for example.

HEAT STROKE

See also: Heat Exhaustion and Sunburn

Heat stroke can be life-threatening and immediate medical help must be sought. Move the child out of the heat and into the shade right away. While waiting for help to arrive, try to get started on lowering the body's temperature. With heat stroke, the body's heat regulation system has stopped working and caused the body temperature to rise. It can happen in extreme heat, when the body fails to adjust to the high temperature, the sweat glands fail to function properly, and the body cannot cool itself down.

Signs and Symptoms

- red hot skin — could be sweaty, or dry
- high temperature
- dizziness, headache, vomiting
- drowsiness — could lead to confusion, and unconsciousness
- the child could have the sensation of being cold, and shiver
- rapid pulse
- body aches and muscular cramps

If possible immerse the child's body in cool to tepid water — not cold. Sponge water over the body. Alternatively, stand the child in a luke-warm shower, and gradually reduce the temperature of the water until it's cool — but not cold. Use any available cool water, even a garden hose — but make the water a very fine spray by applying thumb pressure over the hose exit-hole; and have the child sit down.

Use whatever means you have available to continuously cool the child. Wrap them in cool, wet sheets. If there is a fan at hand, fan the child's face. Cool the child with these different methods, until their temperature is down to 99 degrees. Then cover them with a dry bed sheet. Throughout the cooling process, give them small sips of cool water (see Dehydration).

Baths	*Sponging*
Use cool — not cold — water, and add: *4 drops lavender* *4 drops eucalyptus radiata*	*Sponge the body down with cool to tepid water. Put 1 drop eucalyptus radiata on a sponge, then fill the sponge with water. Start sponging the back of the body first, starting at the back of the neck. Do not sponge the face.*

Essential Oils That Help

Lavender	Eucalyptus radiata
Spearmint	Lemon
Tangerine	Camomile roman
Camomile german	

When to Get Help

Get help immediately if you suspect your child has heat stroke. In the meantime, while waiting for help to arrive, try to start getting the temperature lowered.

Prevention

In hot weather:

- Make sure your child is always wearing a hat and their shoulders are covered.
- Keep your child out of the sun as much as possible.
- Make sure your child has plenty to drink. Water is best.

If running or doing sports:

- Make sure your child has periods of rest. If you're out in the sun, bring them into the shade, and cool them down.
- Make sure your child has plenty to drink. Water is best.

HERPES (GENITAL)

See also: Cold Sores

Most young children with herpes simplex 2 contracted it because their mothers had it, and the virus was passed to them during birth. Herpes simplex 2 is basically a blister-like cold sore on and around the genital area or mouth. Although it's embarrassing, inconvenient, and painful at times, it usually goes away in a week or so.

Genital herpes usually reappears at the same place on the body where the first contact occurred. The herpes simplex 2 infection is usually thought of as entirely genital-area occurrence, but I know from clinical experience that people suffer herpes blisters on other parts of their body too, such as the stomach, buttocks, arms and legs.

The first signs of infection are often flu-like symptoms, with fever, aches and pains, or headache. These go, and are followed by small blisters around the affected area. Infection is spread through the fluid in the blisters. The blisters usually disappear after a week or so, but it can re-erupt at any time. Some people experience outbreaks often, while with others it is seldom. Some people only have the initial outbreak with no other in their lifetime. Home treatment aims to reduce the frequency of outbreaks.

Herpes simplex 2 can be triggered by the same things as cold sores, such as heat or stress. (See Cold Sores.) But because herpes in genital area can't always be exposed to the air, it sometimes takes longer for healing to take place there.

When a child has contracted herpes through their mother, at birth, there may be no visible signs of infection. Such children need to be monitored throughout childhood, and if you are a parent or caretaker, ask your child's doctor what repercussions are likely for your child.

Signs and Symptoms

- tingling, pain, or swelling in the affected area, followed by:
- blisters, that go in time and can reappear

Scientific studies have proven that melissa has an effect on herpes. This is one of the most expensive essential oils, and is often difficult to find. Most essential oil suppliers sell a product called "melissa-type" oil, and not the true melissa you need.

Bathing Methods	
If the essential oil drops touch an open blister, it may sting temporarily. This will not harm your child, and a small amount of Vaseline over the area will neutralize the effect.	
Simple Wash	**Sitz Bath**
Add 2 drops melissa and 2 drops geranium essential oil to a pint of water and bathe the area as often as possible. Swish the water around before using.	The sitz bath method involves putting the child's bottom in a large washing bowl of warm water. First mix the following essential oils: 10 drops tea tree 6 drops lavender 5 drops geranium Put 4 drops of the mix in a large plastic bowl of warm water. Then add: 1 tablespoon salt 1 tablespoon bicarbonate of soda Swish the water around well before your child sits in. Repeat at least three times a day.

Warm Compress Method
To help ease the pain, make disposable compresses by using paper towels. Use a bowl of warm water, adding 5 drops of an essential oil. Use one of the following: camomile german lemon geranium melissa

Essential Oils That Help

Melissa (only if true melissa)	Geranium
Thyme linalol	Tea tree
Manuka	Lemon
Lavender	Camomile german

Other Care

Have your child wear loose clothing in the area of the infection. Growing your own melissa/lemon balm is a good way to get additional help when true melissa is not available, by making an infusion of the leaves, to bathe the area.

When to Get Help

Get a proper medical diagnosis if you suspect your child has genital herpes.

Prevention

- Teach children of all ages to wash hands after visiting any bathroom facility.
- Encourage sexually active teenagers to use condoms.
- If your child has cold sores around their mouth or nose (herpes simplex 1), make sure they understand they should not touch the cold sores and then touch the genital area — as this may lead to cross infection.

While blisters are present:

- Pat the area dry — do not rub.
- The child should always wash their hands with soap after touching sores or blisters.
- No one, including teenagers, should engage in sexual activity while the blisters are present.

HIVES — URTICARIA

Certain raised white lumps, or welts, on the skin are known as hives. There are many reasons why they occur, including contact with certain plants, insect bites, and food allergies. Urticaria is a sensitivity to certain substances which cause the allergic reaction — mostly on the skin, although internal organs can also be affected.

The cause of the hives is often quite obvious — the child has been in contact with a plant, for example, such as nettles or poison ivy, or has been bitten by an insect, such as fire ants, yellow jackets, wasps, bees and hornets. But sometimes the hives appear in response to something consumed, such as shellfish, eggs, nuts, cheese, strawberries, additives, or preservatives. Another less obvious cause is an allergic reaction to medication, such as aspirin, penicillin, or eye drops. Some children develop hives as a result of a minor bacterial, viral, fungal, or yeast infection — including a strep infection of the nose or throat; or from emotional stress such as anger or fear. Other children may develop hives in response to the sun and heat, from exercise, or even from an allergic reaction to the material in a chair they have been sitting on!

It's important to try and identify what your child is allergic to so you can try and prevent further contact. As hives is an allergic reaction, watch your child's face, mouth, and tongue to make sure there is no swelling. If there is, your child may need immediate antihistamine treatment.

Signs and Symptoms

- raised welts on skin — with defined edges that appear raised; white lumps with red surround; blister-like weals
- welts all sizes and shapes; usually confined to one area however, depending on what caused them; can disappear and reappear elsewhere
- stinging, burning sensation at site of welts; intense itchiness
- swelling in area can last up to five days
- headache, feeling unwell, listlessness, cramps
- if face is swollen it may indicate angioneurotic edema (a very serious condition caused by allergy), can cause tongue to swell and requires immediate medical care

Hives are very irritating, and sleep is one of the best remedies. You can gently rub the child's feet to calm them down, and eventually, they will fall asleep.

The bath method is more practical when the hives are scattered over different parts of the body.

Hives Mix

The following combination of essential oils can be used in compresses and baths. First make up the following:

5 drops camomile german
5 drops lavender

From this, use the number of drops recommended in the methods below.

Compress	Baths
Use a cool compress to help soothe the area. Add 2–3 drops of the hives mix to the compress water.	The bath method is more practical when the hives are scattered over different parts of the body. The temperature of the water should be warm — not hot. Add 2–3 drops of the hives mix to the bath water. Adding baking soda to the water will also help, particularly if the hives were caused by an insect bite. Use 1 tablespoon baking soda per bath.

Bedtime Oil

At bedtime, very gently put a small amount of the following oil over the affected area. Mix the following together:

$1/_2$ ounce almond oil
3 drops camomile german
4 drops lavender
2 drops helichrysum
2 drops ormenis flower (camomile maroc)
Mix the essential oils first, then add to the almond oil.

Essential Oils That Help

Camomile german   Ormenis flower (camomile maroc)
Camomile roman   Helichrysum
Lavender

Other Care

Calamine lotion can help soothe the skin. Add 4 drops of lavender and 4 drops of camomile german to 1 ounce calamine lotion.

When to Get Help

Get immediate medical help if your child has difficulty breathing, or if there is any swelling — particularly around the face, mouth, or tongue. Antihistamines should be given at the first sign of swelling, or if the hives get worse. Get help if your child is in pain, or if the hives do not disappear after 24 hours.

Prevention

- There are many possible causes of hives and not much you can do to prevent them on the first occasion. What you can do is to try and prevent further attacks.
- If an insect is the cause, be extra vigilant where they are concerned.
- After the first attack, if there is no obvious plant or insect that caused the hives, make a note of all foods your child ate, medications they took, exercise, stress, and weather details. If there is an obvious cause, try to avoid it in the future. If the cause is uncertain, keep your notes for future reference. If a second attack occurs, you may be able to see similarities between the two occurances.
- If you feel medication was a possible cause, contact your doctor immediately.

IMPETIGO

Impetigo is a highly contagious, skin infection caused by the bacteria staphylococcus and streptococcal. It mainly affects smaller children, and is more common in the summer months. Impetigo is a small rash that can, at its worst turn into a pus-filled sore. It usually appears around the mouth or nose first, but can occur anywhere on the body. It's easily spread by contact. Or, it can even be picked up if a child falls down in the school play yard, skins their knee, and doesn't have the injury looked after properly. If an infected child scratches the area, the bacteria can be transferred to the fingers and spread to other parts of the body, or to other children.

Signs and Symptoms
- small rash with blister-like spots, usually around nose or mouth at first — sometimes mistaken for cold sores
- blisters sometimes filled with pus, becoming open, weeping sores
- sores turn crusty, then a scab forms — and eventually falls off

Wash the affected area thoroughly with soap and water. Use a disposable cloth you can throw away afterwards. Bathing with warm water, and the use of compresses, can give relief. You could use kitchen-roll paper to bathe the area, and a new piece to dab it dry. Take all measures to prevent cross-infection, including taking care to wash your own hands with anti-bacterial soap after carrying out home care measures.

Impetigo Mix

Use the following mix in the tea-dab, and oil methods. First mix these essential oils:

15 drops ravensara
10 drops thyme linalol
15 drops tea tree
10 drops manuka (if not available, substitute an extra 10 drops of tea tree)

Tea-Dab	Oil
After bathing, dab over the area with the following tea. Use the whole mix above in 2 ounces water. Lavender and melissa hydrolats are very useful when used to bathe affected areas. If you have these hydrolats, use them instead of water in the above tea.	Use the whole mix above in $^1/_4$ ounce sesame oil. Blend well, and apply a small amount on affected areas only. Use between bathing.

Compress Method

To 1 dessertspoon of melissa or lavender hydrolat/water, add 1 drop camomile german. Use to soak the compress, and apply over the affected area.

Essential Oils That Help

Ravensara   Thyme linalol
Manuka   Tea tree
Lavender   Niaouli
Camomile german

Other Care

See Prevention, below.

When to Get Help

If you suspect impetigo, see your doctor for a firm diagnosis.

Prevention

- Avoid contact with children who have the infection.

If your child is infected:

- Keep the child's fingernails short to prevent the spread of the infection.
- The child, and all other members of the family, should wash with anti-bacterial soap.
- Take measures to stop the itching.
- Make sure the child uses separate washcloths, towels, and linen.
- Change pillow cases every day to prevent the infection spreading to other parts of the face.
- Although it is common to send infected children to school with impetigo covered, this may not always stop an infection from spreading. It may be advisable to keep the child out of school if they have the infection. Please check with the child's school, for their policy on contagious infections.

INFLUENZA (FLU)

The term flu is given to various strains of the same airborne influenza virus, that cause more or less the same type of symptoms. It can last anywhere from 24 hours to 2 weeks, depending on the strain of the virus. Each strain causes a particular set of symptoms, with some causing more sore throats, for example, while another will seem to have more of an effect on the muscles. All will pass eventually, but home treatment with essential oils will cut down the time of suffering, and aid a full recovery.

Signs and Symptoms

- muscular aches and pains
- headache
- sore throat, cough
- high temperature and fever, and can often include shivering and feeling cold
- red eyes, runny nose
- weakness, tiredness, irritability, crying
- in some cases: vomiting and/or diarrhea

If one member of the household has the flu, diffuse or spray antiviral essential oils in the atmosphere to try and keep cross infection down.

Children Up to 3 Years of Age

Apply the following mix to the back, and upper chest:

1 teaspoon almond oil
1 drop thyme linalol
2 drops ravensara

Children Over 4 Years of Age

Only use this method if you have these essential oils available:

thyme linalol (no other type of thyme can be substituted)
ravensara

First open both bottles of oil. Put 1 drop thyme linalol in the palm of one hand, and add to it, 1 drop ravensara. Rub your hands together and rub over the child's back. Then immediately smooth over the same area using $^1/_4$–$^1/_2$ teaspoon vegetable oil. Do the same thing on the child's upper chest.

Warning: *This is one of the few times the professional method of using essential oils directly on the skin is recommended for home use, but ensure you only use the essential oils listed above.*

Body Massage

Make a massage oil by mixing:

$^1/_4$ *ounce almond oil*
5 drops thyme linalol
5 drops ravensara
Use 1 teaspoon of the above mix to massage the arms and legs, as well as the neck, back, and front. Avoid the genital area.

Nighttime Methods

Diffuser Spray

Before your child goes to sleep, diffuse the following essential oils in their room:

2 drops thyme linalol
2 drops oregano
2 drops cinnamon
2 drops clove
Alternatively, use 8 drops of one of the following mixes:

Influtect*
Dermatect*
Bronchotect*

If using a diffuser make sure it is not left in their room overnight.

*See Suppliers

Pillow

At least one hour before the child goes to bed, put several drops of thyme linalol on their pillow — under a corner, away from their eyes.

Essential Oils That Help

Ravensara   Thyme linalol

Eucalyptus radiata   Niaouli

Other Care

Children get bored and miserable when they have the flu, so keep your child near you during the day by making up a bed on the sofa. What they need most now is kind, loving attention — and plenty of rest. Try to reduce any fever with the compress method. Avoid giving milk products as they increase mucus within the body. Give small drinks of pure fruit juice, and lots of water.

When to Get Help

Get medical advice if your child is asthmatic, diabetic, or has a weakened immune system. Flu symptoms are similar to those of other infections and diseases, so watch to make sure your child does not develop a rash. If the child does develop a rash, consult your doctor immediately. Also get medical help if the child complains of an earache, if the cough gets worse, or if the temperature does not go down after 36 hours.

Prevention

The flu is all too easy to catch and there's not much you can do to prevent it. But you can try to stop the flu spreading to other members of the family.

- If other members of the family are at home, keep the child with flu in bed and isolated from others.
- Dispose of used tissues in a closed bin immediately after use.
- Use Antiinfectious Air Spray on page 37.

INGROWN TOENAILS

When the side of a toenail becomes imbedded in the surrounding tissue, instead of growing straight out, it is said to be "ingrown." A nail might grow into the tissue because of a natural curve or, more likely, because poor fitting shoes have forced it in that direction. Shoes that are too narrow across the toes are often to blame.

Signs and Symptoms
- usually big toe is affected
- area around ingrown toenail very sore, and particularly painful when walking
- tissue around ingrown toenail red and swollen
- can become infected

Foot Bath

Soaking the toes in water softens the nails. Adding the following essential oils to the water, may help to avoid the area becoming infected. Soak the affected area at least twice a day. To a foot bath add:

1 teaspoon salt
1 teaspoon Epsom salts
1 teaspoon baking soda
2 drops lavender
2 drops tea tree

To Relieve Pain and Prevent Infection

Put 1 drop of the following essential oil mix around the toe area, twice a day:

5 drops lavender
5 drops tea tree

Essential Oils That Help

Lavender	Tea Tree
Helichrysum	Ravensara
Camomile roman	

Other Care

Have your child wear open-toed shoes whenever possible, and go barefoot or in socks when at home.

When to Get Help

A doctor or podiatrist will usually be able to remove the embedded section of nail, and dress the toe, although surgery is sometimes required. Even after a toenail has been correctly cut, it can still become inflamed. If your child develops a temperature, or if you see any sign of a white mass under the nail, get medical attention because there could be an infection. When you first suspect your child might have an ingrown toenail, and even if it's not very painful, get medical advice. It's important to deal with this problem now, to prevent difficulties in later life.

Prevention

- Ingrown toenails are often an on-going problem, so check on the nails as they grow, and take prompt action if it happens again.
- Make sure your child's shoes are not too tight — width, as well as in length.

LARYNGITIS

Laryngitis is a mild inflammation of the larynx, the vocal chords, and voice box. It can last up to a week and is not generally serious except, potentially, for babies and small children. Laryngitis can be caused by viral and bacterial infection, allergy, irritation from a smoky atmosphere, or using the voice too much. Professional singers are prone to laryngitis, as are people who shout loudly at sporting events. Laryngitis is more common during the fall and winter months, when many cold and flu viruses seem to be around.

Signs and Symptoms
- sore throat, hoarse voice
- difficulty in swallowing, breathing difficulties
- dry cough
- fever, tiredness, generally feeling not well
- a baby sounds hoarse when it cries, possible loss of voice
- larynx becomes swollen and obstructs airways of smaller infants
- can lead to croup in smaller infants

Laryngitis is a common problem, and people have found many natural ways to help ease the symptoms. An opera singer once told me that she and her colleagues relied on canned peaches in syrup — they either ate the peaches, or put them through a blender and sipped on them all day. Apparently it worked wonderfully.

Keeping the air moist is very helpful, and this can be done using a humidifier, room spray, or bowls of steaming water. Baths and showers also provide moist air for a short time. Essential oils can be used in all these methods: see pages 15–24 for directions on how to prepare the different methods and for the number of drops of essential oil to use for children of different ages; see the Essential Oils That Help or Laryngitis Mix below.

Laryngitis Mix

The following mix can be used in the Soothing Oil and Cool Compress methods below. Follow the directions in each box. First mix together:

5 drops camomile german
5 drops ravensara
2 drops helichrysum

Soothing Oil Mix

Add the laryngitis mix to 1 ounce vegetable oil. Use a small amount each time. Gently apply over the front of the neck.

Cool Compress

Add 3 drops of the laryngitis mix above to a small bowl of cool — not cold — water. Soak a compress in the water, squeeze out, and apply over the front of the neck.

Laryngitis Tea

Only a small amount of this tea is used each time.

Put three lemons, and a handful of fresh mint if you have it, into a tea pot and cover with $1/2$ pint boiling water. Add 1 tablespoon honey, and stir before replacing the lid. Leave to cool. Then add 1 drop lemon essential oil, stir again, and pour through an unbleached paper coffee filter.

Children over 5 years of age can sip 1 tablespoon of the tea slowly.
For children under 5 years of age, dilute 1 tablespoon of the tea in 1 tablespoon water, and sip slowly.

Essential Oils That Help

Ravensara
Ginger
Eucalyptus radiata
Cajeput

Camomile german
Thyme linalol
Helichrysum
Geranium

Other Care

Give the child plenty of soothing, warm — but not hot — drinks, such as warm water and honey; warm water, honey, and lemon; warm water and fruit juice. To allow the throat inflammation to calm down, stop your child from shouting or talking a lot. That will only make the hoarse voice worse. Allow fresh air in the home, and keep the atmosphere moist.

When to Get Help

Babies and infants with laryngitis need to be closely watched to make sure the larynx does not become swollen and obstruct the airways. Should this occur, immediate medical attention must be sought. If the laryngitis develops into croup (see Croup), see your physician as soon as possible. Also seek medical advice if your child develops a high temperature, or if you suspect there may be an infection other than laryngitis.

LYME DISEASE

Lyme disease is caused by a microorganism carried by a tic that usually lives on deer. Infection can occur if a person is bitten by one of these deer tics, although the disease is not transmitted unless the tic has remained attached to the skin for approximately 24 hours. The tics live in grassy and woodland areas, and are more active during the summer. It's often difficult to realize infection has occurred because the tics are so small and easily overlooked, the bite is not felt, and a rash does not always develop. Lyme disease was only recognized as a specific condition in 1975. A blood test is needed to get a positive diagnosis.

Signs and Symptoms

- when bitten, a circular red rash appears, with a distinct spot in the middle
- the rash clears, leaving a circular mark
- in the weeks following the bite, a rash could occur on other parts of the body
- flu-like symptoms, including fever, headache, muscle ache and pain, listlessness, tiredness, and irritability
- arthritis-like symptoms can develop over time — with swollen and painful joints
- in the worst cases, the central nervous system is affected with numbness, paralysis, and heart problems

Lyme disease is a very serious condition that requires a proper diagnosis and medical treatment. Essential oils can help as a deterrent — to stop tics from coming near your child. Also, after being bitten, if you are camping and far away from medical facilities, essential oils can be used as emergency treatment until you can get medical help.

Deterrent Clothing Spray

If you are going into an area where deer live and the tic may be present, prepare the following mix and take it with you. Store it in a spray bottle. Spray clothing — especially around the neck line, cuffs, the hems of skirts or bottoms of trouser legs, on shoes, socks, and the outside of hats. Allow to dry, then repeat.

In a small bowl, first mix the following:

30 drops citronella
30 drops lemongrass
20 drops eucalyptus radiata
10 drops peppermint
10 drops niaouli

Then add $1/4$ ounce neem oil — if available, but beware, it has a very strong smell. (Neem comes from India — ask in Asian shops. It can also be found in some health food stores.) Next, pour 8 ounces hot water onto the mix, and put a plate over the bowl so the condensed steam water is caught in the mix when the water cools. Let stand for at least 48 hours. Finally, strain the mix through an unbleached paper coffee filter and bottle.

Neat Oils — Clothing Deterrent Mix

Make up a mix, using the same essential oils listed in the clothing spray above. Put 1–2 drops on socks, trouser bottoms, hems, shirt cuffs, shirt collars, and around the brim of hats.

Use on the clothing of children who are 7 years of age or older.

For children under 7 years of age, use neat niaouli and eucalyptus radiata essential oil, in the same method as above. An alternative deterrent is lavender oil, but try to avoid that if you regularly use it to help your child sleep.

Deterrent Body Massage Oil

This body massage may help prevent your child being bitten. It can be used during the night, or in the day. It can also be used on children who have already been bitten. Rub the oil all over the body. This is enough for several applications. Mix together:

1 tablespoon vegetable oil
2 drops niaouli
3 drops lavender

Emergency Care

If your child has been bitten and you are camping far from medical help, put a couple of drops of whatever essential oil you have with you, neat, directly on the bite, before extracting the tic with tweezers. Then wash the bite thoroughly with soap and water, and put 1 drop of neat lavender or thyme linalol directly on the bite. Try to get help as soon as possible.

In the meantime, repeat the wash and neat essential oil application at least once a day, and use the body massage method on the child as well.

Using essential oils as insect deterrents has become very popular. The list below contains essential oils that are suitable for use on children's clothing. As these will be used while hiking or camping, I assume the child will not be wearing any expensive, delicate clothing, as some of these essential oils may leave a mark on the material.

Essential Oils That Help

To Deter Tics:	To Ease a Tic Bite:	With the Rash:
Lavender	Thyme Linalol	Camomile german
Eucalyptus radiata	Niouli	Lavender
Peppermint		
Thyme Linalol		
Lemongrass		
Citronella		
Palmarosa		

When to Get Help

Call a doctor immediately if you suspect that your child has been bitten, as early treatment prevents damage in later life.

Prevention

Prevention is much better than cure. Take precautions if your child is playing in long grass or woods where deer live.

- Have your child wear long sleeves and trousers, and tuck the trouser legs into socks. Put a hat on your child, and have them wear light colored clothing.
- Check your child for any tiny tics — look in the hair lines, as well as more obvious places.
- If you see a tic, remove it very carefully with tweezers and apply disinfectant to the area. To make a correct diagnosis easier, take the tic with you to a doctor.
- If you take a pet into the area, check them for tics also.

MEASLES — RUBEOLA

Measles is a highly contagious, airborne, viral infection, that is spread through coughing and sneezing. After exposure to the virus, the incubation period is approximately 10 to 14 days. Although measles immunization is mandatory in most U.S. schools, cases do still occur. Most affected children go through the infection with no bad side effects, but measles is potentially very dangerous because it makes a child vulnerable to other infections such as bronchitis and pneumonia, and to ear infections which can lead to deafness.

Signs and Symptoms
- begins with cold-like symptoms: runny nose, cough, fever, listlessness
- small red spots with white centers, on the tissue lining the inside of the mouth
- itchy rash appears 2 to 4 days after the spots in the mouth — starts at the forehead, spreads over the face, neck, behind the ears, then over the tummy, and to other areas of the body
- eyes red and sore, and sensitive to bright light
- respiratory difficulties
- may also have abdominal pain, vomiting, or diarrhea

There are many approaches to aromatherapy measles management, including baths and sponging to soothe the rash and aid recovery, the humidifier method for coughs that do not ease, rest for the body, compresses for sore eyes, and diffusers and other room methods to prevent the infection from spreading.

Soothing Baths

Oat Bath	Oil Bath	Bicarbonate Soda Bath
Put a handful of raw oats or oatmeal in a piece of material, and add to it:	Put 1 tablespoon sea salt in the bath water. Then dilute the following essential oils in 1 teaspoon vegetable oil:	Mix the following essential oils in 1 cup bicarbonate of soda:
4 drops camomile german 4 drops lavender 4 drops ravensara	1 drops lavender 2 drops bergamot 3 drops tea tree	2 drops lavender 1 drops camomile german 4 drops geranium
Tie the bundle securely, then attach it to the water faucet of the bath, so the water can run through the bundle before reaching the bath.	Also add to the bath. Swish the water around well before the child gets in.	Mix the essential oils in thoroughly with a spoon. Then add to the bath water.

Sponging Method

First mix the following:

5 drops bergamot
5 drops camomile german
5 drops lavender

Use 5 drops for each sponge down to help reduce fever. Put tepid or warm — not hot — water in a small bowl and add 5 drops of the essential oil mix. Swish the water around, then soak a sponge or wash cloth in it, squeeze it out, and use to sponge down the whole of your child's body — avoiding the face and genital area.

Humidifier	Rest	Eye Compress
If your child has a cough that does not ease, use essential oils from the Essential Oils That Help list in humidifiers and steaming baths .	To help the child get a good night's sleep put a drop or two of camomile roman or lavender on a corner of their pillow — on the underside, away from eyes. If neither of these help, try neroli essential oil, which is sometimes effective when the others are not.	If your child's eyes are sore, place a cool wet cloth over them. You can also make a camomile roman tea, or a camomile hydrolat and use one of them for the compress water. Make sure you squeeze the compress out well, and that your child keeps their eyes closed.

Preventative Atmosphere
To help prevent the spread of infection, use the vaporizer, diffuser, or water spray method. Mix the following essential oils: 10 drops bergamot 20 drops ravensara 10 drops geranium Use 4–6 drops each time. If you do not have these essential oils, use any on the Essential Oils That Help list that follows.

Essential Oils That Help

Camomile german   Lavender
Niaouli   Ravensara
Thyme linalol   Cajeput
Eucalyptus radiata   Tea tree
Bergamot

Other Care

Your child must stay in bed, and be kept away from other children, even if they have been immunized. Adults can also catch measles and, as with many other so-called "childhood" diseases, it can be far worse for adults. Make sure you take all possible precautions to avoid catching the infection yourself.

When to Get Help

If you suspect measles, consult your child's doctor immediately. If your child recovers from measles, and then gets worse again, possibly with an earache, consult the doctor again. Inform your child's school that he/she has measles, so other parents can be told to watch for signs and symptoms in their children.

Prevention

- Immunization is mandatory in most U.S. schools, and although this has certainly stopped the spread of this potentially dangerous infection, doubts have been raised as to the total safety of the vaccine. If your child is allergic to eggs, tell your doctor because the measles vaccine is developed on eggs, and this may cause a reaction in your child.

MENARCHE — MENSTRUAL PROBLEMS

Menarche is the onset of the menstrual cycle. The average age that a girl starts her period is between the ages of 11 and 13. Some girls, however, start as early as 8, while others may find themselves waiting until they're 17 or 18.

Signs and Symptoms
- uterine cramps
- backache
- flow can be light or heavy
- the first flow can be very dark

It's important to prepare your daughter for the onset of menarche, by giving her sanitary napkins, showing her how to use them, and telling her it will start unexpectedly with a feeling of wetness and/or discomfort.

Girls often feel embarrassed about menstruation and don't want fathers or brothers to know they've started. Be sensitive to your daughter's wishes about this, because if you betray her trust on this important occasion, she may be less inclined to confide in you during her later teens — perhaps over issues you may need to know about.

Tummy Rub

Geranium essential oil is a blessing for women of all ages, as it is a great help in dealing with cramps and blood flow problems.

Put 4 drops neat geranium oil on the tummy, over the uterine area, and spread it around. Then cover this area with a small amount of vegetable oil.

Let your daughter sit and rest with something warm over the area. If you use a hot water bottle, use warm — not hot — water; or use the type of bag that can be heated in a microwave.

Warm Baths

The following essential oil bath can help with all the symptoms of menstruation, plus lessen any anxiety your daughter may be feeling. Mix together:

1 teaspoon vegetable oil
3 drops geranium
1 drops bergamot
2 drops lavender

Pour the mixture into the bath, as the warm water is running. Tell your daughter that if she finds globules of oil floating on the water, scoop them into her hand and rub the oil into her skin, over her tummy. If her breasts are sore, she can massage the floating oil into them as well.

Essential Oils That Help

Geranium	Rose
Lavender	Camomile roman
Helichrysum	

When to Get Help

Medical help is not usually required when girls start their menstruation, however, you should seek advice if: your daughter's cramps are so bad she can't move without pain; if she has pain urinating or defecating; or if she has severe premenstrual syndrome (PMS).

MENINGITIS

Meningitis is caused by several different types of bacteria and virus, and leads to inflammation of the meninges — the lining of the brain. Meningitis is spread by an infected person sneezing, coughing or kissing, or by poor hygiene, or unsanitary water.

The bacterial types of meningitis can be life threatening if not detected early enough, while the viral types are much less severe. Early diagnosis is the key to treating meningitis and if you have any suspicion your child has this infection, do not wait for help, but take your child right away to the nearest medical facility and demand that they are seen immediately.

The difficulty with meningitis is that the early symptoms are very much like those of the flu. This can confuse doctors, as well as parents. The symptoms of both bacterial and viral meningitis are similar to begin with, and the illness can develop over a couple of days. However, in serious cases, there will come a point when the child suddenly gets worse.

If your child has symptoms of meningitis, it's important to find out which type it is. The viral types of meningitis are much more common — and much less dangerous — than the bacterial type. If you suspect meningitis, go to the nearest hospital and have tests to ascertain which type your child has. Antibiotics cannot fight viral meningitis, and treatment for this type usually just consists of good nursing care.

Bacterial meningitis is the one everyone worries about. There are two types: meningococcal and pneumococcal. The first symptoms usually appear 2 to 10 days after infection. Most children will make a full recovery, if diagnosis and treatment are given early. However, bacterial meningitis can lead to deafness, brain damage, or even death. Children of all ages are at risk, including newborn babies.

The symptom lists refer to the most usual symptoms. An affected child might just have one of these symptoms, or many.

Signs and Symptoms

In babies:

- fever, yet hands and feet might feel cold and look blue
- blank, staring expression
- may refuse food, or vomit
- may be difficult to wake up, baby has no energy
- fontanel — the soft spot on the top of the skull — may feel tense, or bulge
- makes strange noises — whimpering, or a high-pitched moan
- does not like to be picked up
- neck retraction: the head is pushing backwards, often with arched back
- skin is pale or blotchy

In children:

- symptoms may seem similar to those of the flu
- stiff neck
- high temperature, fever
- severe headache
- vomiting
- pain in joints or muscles
- sensitivity to bright light
- seizure
- drowsiness, lethargy
- small purplish-red rash, that can still be seen when a glass is pressed against it
- rashes anywhere on the body

One of the symptoms of meningitis is neck pain. Don't just ask your child if their neck hurts, they are likely to say yes even if they only have the flu. Gently take your child's head in your hands and try to move it. First, move it forward, then backward, then to one side, then the other. If the child now says the neck hurts, or if the neck cannot move, then meningitis may be present.

Another symptom of meningitis is joint or muscle pain. If the child complains of pains in their leg, or a smaller child volunteers a leg hurt, this might indicate meningitis. Sensitivity to light is a classic symptom of meningitis —

bring a table lamp to the child, or use a flash light if nothing else is available, and watch the child's reaction closely. They may squint their eyes, or whimper, or pull away. Babies with meningitis have the symptom of disliking being picked up or handled. This is very unusual for a baby, especially if they are ill with something less severe than meningitis. Take this symptom seriously. Also, with a baby, feel the top of their head, in the fontanel region: if it bulges or feels hard, this is a classic symptom of meningitis.

The characteristic rash that accompanies some forms of meningitis — particularly the bacterial meningococcal strain — shows that blood poisoning (septicemia) has taken place. If you get a clear glass and press it against a meningitis rash, the rash stays clearly visible through the glass. With most other rashes, when you press a glass against it, the rash will temporarily fade.

Meningitis is a life-threatening disease and requires immediate medical treatment. Although there are essential oils with antibacterial and antiviral properties it is only appropriate at this time to use essential oils to soothe the child, and help with some of the symptoms. Choose from the methods on pages 15–31, using the number of drops recommended for the different age groups.

The viral types of meningitis are treated with good nursing care, and this is where essential oils can really help. Use essential oils in baths, and in hand and foot massages — don't massage the whole body. Room sprays are useful at this time, as they can lift the spirits of a sick child, cheer them up slightly, and offer protection against cross-infection. Essential oils used in the water-spray method, over your child's bed linen, can help freshen up that area. A combination of essential oils that is a favorite with children, and would help cheer them up at this time, is equal parts of geranium and orange.

Essential Oils That Help

The following essential oils can be used alongside conventional medical treatment, and used to help lessen the symptoms of meningitis. For the appropriate dosage — the number of drops to use — see page 24.

Camomile roman	Camomile german
Lavender	Ormenis flower (*Camomile Maroc*)
Cardamom	Palmarosa
Ravensara	Niaouli

Other Care

Give your child plenty of fluid to drink, especially water.

When to Get Help

Always get immediate emergency help if you suspect meningitis.

Prevention

- Speak to your physician about immunization. There are vaccines for some forms of meningitis, including bacterial haemophilus influenza type b (Hib).
- Be especially vigilant if your child has recently had another type of illness, such as mumps, a throat infection, or the flu, as meningitis sometimes erupts after having these.
- If meningitis has been diagnosed in other children in your area, keep your child away from all children, as much as possible.
- If your child has meningitis, inform their school right away, so other parents can look for symptoms in their children.

MIGRAINE

A migraine is an attack of severe pain and continual ache in the head. There are different types of migraine — some cause nausea and sickness, or make a child shield their eyes from light, while others do not. Migraine might run in the family, or not. Each individual has different triggers — it may be stress or anxiety, computer overuse, perfumes, pollutants, bright lights, being in a stuffy atmosphere, or eating a food they are allergic to. Classic culprits are cheese, caffeine in sodas, chocolate, oranges, tomatoes, and spicy foods. Each child will have an individual profile of causes of migraine, and an individual symptom profile that may include some or all of those below.

Signs and Symptoms

- head pain and ache — often over one eye and one side of face
- disturbed vision, eye ache
- seeing strange colors around objects
- pale skin tone
- abdominal pain, neckache
- tingling and other unusual sensations in body
- numb feeling in head and face
- abnormal sense of smell — either loss of smell or heightened smell

---

Cold Compresses

Cold compresses can give some relief. Put 1 pint cold water in a small bowl and add:

3 drops grapefruit
2 drops lavender

Put a light cloth in the bowl, squeeze out well, and place on the back of the child's neck, or on the forehead, making sure the compress is well squeezed out. Put the unused compress water in the refrigerator to keep cool, and use it to refresh the compress during the migraine attack.

General Migraine Body Massage

First blend the following essential oils:

5 drops camomile roman
10 drops grapefruit
5 drops peppermint
3 drops rosemary

If your child is 7 years of age and under, dilute the above in 4 ounces vegetable oil. If your child is 8 years of age or over, dilute in $1^1/_2$ ounces vegetable oil.

Use a small amount of the diluted oil in a massage for at least 15 minutes, once a week. Take the phone off the hook, and have the child lay on their front. Gently massage their back, shoulders, legs, and arms, always working toward the direction of the heart.

Nausea Tummy Rub

If the child suffers from nausea and sickness during a migraine attack, prepare the essential oil mix as for the General Migraine Body Massage, and instead of massaging the whole body, you could just rub a little of the diluted oil over the child's abdomen, and the back of their neck.

Stress Migraine Body Massage

This massage oil is helpful if the child's migraine is brought on by stress. Use equal amounts of the essential oils of:

neroli
petitgrain

See page 31 for the appropriate number of drops of essential oil to use for the age of your child. Dilute the appropriate number of drops of essential oil in vegetable oil.
Use a small amount of diluted oil in a body massage for at least 15 minutes, once or twice a week. Take the phone off the hook, and have your child lay on their front. Gently massage the back, shoulders, legs, and arms, always working toward the direction of the heart.

Regular gentle massage will help to keep your child less stressed, and introduce a parent's loving touch.

Essential Oils That Help

Grapefruit	Lavender
Camomile roman	Neroli
Petitgrain	Marjoram
Peppermint	Rosemary

Other Care

Lie your child down on a bed or sofa, pull the curtains to darken the room, make sure there is a window open, to air the room. Your child may feel sick, so put a bucket nearby they can be sick into. Your child will feel worse if they have to run to the bathroom to be sick, should the need arise.

Give your child plenty of liquids; grapefruit juice has been known to be helpful in lessening the severity of the attack in some children. Make sure your child has eaten. Migraine often comes on if your child has skipped lunch or breakfast. If they have, give them something light to eat. Even if your child feels sick and says they don't want anything, they may feel better if they eat. Then your child needs quiet, rest, and sleep.

When to Get Help

See your physician if your child complains of stomach pains or has recurring migraine attacks.

Prevention

- Keep a diary to try and find out what causes the migraine. Write down all foods and drinks consumed prior to the attack, what subjects were coming up on your child's school agenda, who came to visit your home, and where your child visited. Try to eliminate the triggers. It may be that certain people or places make your child stressed or anxious. Your child may be having an allergic reaction to a chemical or pollutant in the atmosphere. Or, did they spend too long watching television or on the computer? Write everything that happens on the day of the attack, so you can compare notes if it happens again. There are so many possible causes of migraine, all you can do is try to narrow them down. In this way, you may be able to identify triggers to your child's migraine, and avoid them in the future.

MONONUCLEOSIS (MONO, THE KISSING DISEASE)

Mono is a common viral infection, a member of the herpes family, that is caused by the Epstein-Barr virus. It's often transmitted by mouth contact and saliva, which is why it's called "the kissing disease," and why teenagers are usually the group who are affected. However, mono can also be caught by younger children, by breathing in infectious moisture from the air. The symptoms appear around two weeks after infection, and the condition usually clears up within one to four weeks, depending on the child and severity of the infection.

Signs and Symptoms

- flu-like symptoms, aches and pains, generally feeling unwell
- fatigue and overwhelming tiredness
- swollen lymph nodes (glands in the neck)
- sore throat; enlarged tonsils covered with mucus
- high temperature

Back, Chest, and Throat Oil	Warm Baths
The following oil can be rubbed over your child's back, chest, and throat. Mix the essential oils first, then add to the vegetable oil. Use a small amount each time.	Warm baths will help make your child feel better. Add 4 drops of the following mix to 1 teaspoon vegetable oil and add to the bath water.
1 tablespoon vegetable oil 10 drops tea tree 5 drops lemon 10 drops eucalyptus radiata 6 drops ravensara	3 drops ravensara 5 drops mandarin This makes enough for two baths.

Sore Throat Gargle Mix	*Diffuser*
Only use this method if your child is old enough to spit the water out after the gargle. It will help ease a sore throat.	*To help your child sleep well, use the following essential oils in a diffuser in the child's bedroom as they go to sleep.*
First using the tea method, make a tea using lemon and geranium essential oil.	*2 drops lavender*
For the gargle, put the following in a small glass of water:	*1 drop camomile roman* *3 drops mandarin*
1 teaspoon lemon and geranium tea *¹/₂ teaspoon salt* *1 teaspoon vinegar*	*Don't leave the diffuser in the room overnight.*
Stir well, and have the child gargle with this. Make sure they spit it out afterward. Repeat three times a day.	

Essential Oils That Help

Lavender   Ravensara

Niaouli   Cajeput

Camomile roman

Other Care

Give your child plenty of fluid. They should do no strenuous exercise and get plenty of rest.

When to Get Help

Contact your physician if the young person or child develops a high fever, has breathing difficulties, or if the tiredness and weakness continues after the infection has past.

Prevention

- Avoid contact with infected persons.

If your child has mono:

- Keep your child isolated from other members of the household.
- Dispose of all mucus-laden tissues in a closed bin immediately after use.
- Teach your child to cough directly into a tissue, and dispose of it immediately by flushing it down the toilet.

MOTION SICKNESS

Motion sickness can result from travelling in cars, boats, trains, planes, amusement park rides, and even from playground swings. Travel by car is the most common cause of motion sickness, and can be made worse for sensitive children by general road pollution or leakage of fuel fumes from the vehicle itself .

Motion sickness is caused by the delicate mechanism in the inner ear, and the fluids contained in it, becoming out of balance by repeated movement of the head and body. Fast-moving, conflicting messages being received from the eyes to the brain don't help.

In some children, the very thought of having to travel makes them tense and anxious and they begin to get some of the symptoms of motion sickness before they've even stepped outside the front door!

Signs and Symptoms

- vomiting, feeling unwell, feeling faint, dizziness, perspiration
- drowsiness, yawning, breathing more heavily
- a cold, clammy feel to skin, or unusual pallor to skin
- in some cases earache

If the child vomits, give them liquid to ensure they don't get dehydrated.

Babies

Exclude peppermint from blends for babies under 2 years of age, and only use the vehicle tissue method.

◇

Put 1 drop of the motion sickness mix on a tissue and tuck somewhere in the travel vehicle.

◇

Give the baby sips of cooled, boiled water during the journey.

Teas	*Motion Sickness Mix*	*Other*
These methods can only be used on children over 2 years of age. Make up one of the following teas before a planned trip. Cool, bottle, and take it with you. Have the child sip it slowly during the journey. ☙ Make tea with fresh peppermint herb and root ginger. Slice a small piece of fresh ginger and some pieces of fresh mint. Add boiling water, cover, and leave to brew for at least 10 minutes. Bottle when cooled. ☙ Make tea using one peppermint and one ginger tea bag. Cover and leave to brew for ten minutes. Bottle when cooled.	Mix together: 10 drops ginger 4 drops peppermint 2 drops eucalyptus radiata 2 drops coriander Dilute 2 drops of the mixture in 1 teaspoon vegetable oil, and rub a small amount over the child's back and abdomen before the journey starts.	Put one drop of the Motion Sickness Mix on a tissue and tuck it down in the seat behind the child. ☙ Put 4 drops ginger oil on a tissue and sniff as required.

Flying Anxiety

Before traveling: For the younger child, add 1 drop lavender and 1 drop of geranium to a small amount of vegetable oil, and put it in the bath. It will float, and can be collected in the hands and massaged into the child's skin, under the water. An older child can massage it into themselves.

During the flight: Take with you a prepared mix of 5 drops each of chamomile, lavender, and geranium, diluted in one ounce vegetable oil. A younger child will allow you to massage a little of this into their feet, while for older children, place 2 drops lavender onto a tissue and place it behind them, on the seat. Both methods help to calm. If the child feels sick, put 2 drops Motion Sickness Mix on a tissue, for them to sniff.

Essential Oils That Help

Ginger	Rosemary
Peppermint	Coriander
Eucalyptus radiata	Cardamom

Prevention

- Have the child lie down with their eyes closed on the back seat of the car. Ensure the seat belt is used. If this is difficult, have the child lay back in the seat with cushions supporting their head.
- Some children find it easier if they always look directly ahead during car travel.
- It sometimes helps if the child can nibble on dry crackers, or sip water/tea while travelling.
- Open the window to get fresh air; or, if in a traffic jam with the window open, close it to keep pollution out of the vehicle.
- Don't make an issue of motion sickness before travel as this may upset the child and precondition them into actually being sick.

MUMPS

Mumps are caused by an airborne virus that affects the parotid salivary glands. The most characteristic symptom of mumps is large swellings just below the ears. Mumps are usually caught in the same way so many other conditions are — by people sneezing or coughing infected moisture into the air, although direct contact with an infected person's saliva will also transmit the virus. Symptoms appear a couple of weeks after infection and last for a few days. The virus is contagious during the two days before the glands swell and for approximately ten days afterward.

Usually mumps are fairly harmless, but there can be serious complications. In rare cases, the brain can become affected, and meningitis may develop. Occasionally, permanent deafness results from mumps. Sometimes other glands become involved, particularly the testes, ovaries, and pancreas. If your child is a boy, watch to make sure his testicles don't become swollen. If they do, inform your doctor right away. If a boy catches mumps during puberty, it can result in sterility. The same is the case for adult men who did not have mumps as a child.

Signs and Symptoms

- large swelling on one or both sides of the neck (the glands), just below the ears, can be very sore
- difficulty in swallowing, dry mouth
- mild fever
- headache, earache
- sometimes face and tongue are swollen
- in serious cases: painful swollen testicles (boys), or lower abdominal ovarian pain (girls)

Compresses

Essential oils can be used in compresses applied over the swollen glands. Some children prefer warm compresses, others prefer the water to be cool. Older children can be asked which feels best to them. To half a pint of water, add 4 drops of the following mix:

10 drops eucalyptus radiata
5 drops thyme linalol
4 drops lavender

Put the compress in the water, squeeze it out, and apply to both glands in the neck, under the ears.

Back and Neck Oil

First make a mix of essential oils using the following:

15 drops lavender
5 drops camomile roman
5 drops camomile german
5 drops eucalyptus radiata

Dilute the essential oil mix in 1 teaspoon vegetable oil, using the following amount:

Up to 5 years	*3 drops*
6–8 years	*4 drops*
9 years and over	*5 drops*

Use the diluted oil to massage the back. Also apply to the neck without massaging. Do this twice a day.

Baths

Mix the following essential oils:

4 drops lavender
4 drops geranium
4 drops mandarin

Dilute 4 drops of the mix in 1 teaspoon vegetable oil, and add to the bath water. This is enough essential oils mix for 3 baths.

Mumps Mix

The following mix can be used in the Over 7 Method and the Abdominal Rub. Follow directions for each method. First mix the following essential oils together:

5 drops thyme linalol
5 drops lavender
10 drops ravensara

Over 7 Method	Abdominal Rub
Only use this method if your child is over 7 years of age.	Dilute 3 drops of the mumps mix in 1 teaspoon vegetable oil. Smooth over the lower abdomen, avoiding the genital area. Do not use on the testicles.
Apply 1 drop of the mumps mix directly on the swollen gland under the ears. If both sides are swollen, use 1 drop on each side.	
Use this method no more than once a day, at bedtime is best.	

Essential Oils That Help

Tea tree   Coriander
Lemon   Lavender
Camomile roman   Ravensara
Niaouli   Helichrysum
Eucalyptus radiata

Other Care

Give your child plenty of fluid, avoiding citrus fruit juices and other acidic drinks. It can be difficult to swallow easily at this time, so give your child soups, and mashed-up or liquidated foods. Ice cream will help to cool the throat.

Some children get relief by having something warm against their neck, such as a warm towel, warm pack, or hot-water bottle — (warm, not hot). Other children prefer something cool against their neck, such as a cool compress. Ask your child what feels best to them.

When to Get Help

Contact your doctor as soon as you suspect mumps. Call your doctor again if, in the case of a boy, the testicles become swollen or, in the case of a girl, she experiences lower abdominal pain. Your doctor should also be told if your child's neck gets stiff and painful, if there are headaches, or if the condition does not improve within 10 days.

Prevention

- It is possible to be inoculated against mumps. The vaccines are cultured on egg protein, so if your child is allergic to eggs, discuss that with your doctor before proceeding.

MUSCLES — OVEREXERCISED

See also: Strains

Children are supposed to be active, but sometimes they overdo it — playing sports, running, cycling, doing gymnastics, or exercises, too many dance lessons, or just climbing and jumping all day. And overexercised muscles are sometimes the result.

Signs and Symptoms

- aching muscles — sometimes with pain
- usually in legs and arms
- worse in morning
- stiff muscles

When a child has overdone the exercise, or been playing too zealously, the best course of action is to apply a body oil and rub it into the muscles, just before your child has a warm bath. The bath helps the essential oils sink into the skin so they can warm and soothe the muscles. The child should soak in the bath for a while to give their muscles a chance to relax. Give older children a book to read, and younger children a toy to play with. This relaxing routine may give your child an appreciation of relaxing baths, which in later life could provide them with an escape from the stresses of life.

The following massage oil and bath method is not to be used just because your child has been physically active, but because after the activity they complain of muscle ache and are in need of care.

Overexercised Muscles, Pre-Bath Oil Mix

The following routine will reduce the likelihood of sore, stiff muscles in the morning. It is most effective if carried out before bedtime. First mix the following essential oils together:

3 drops marjoram
2 drops camomile roman
2 drops lavender
2 drops ginger

See page 16 for the number of drops of essential oils to dilute in 1 teaspoon vegetable oil, depending on the age-group of your child. Apply enough of the oil to cover the skin over the aching or sore muscles, and rub in. Then let your child have a warm bath, where they should soak and relax.

If your child is very dirty, after a football game for example, they should have a shower before the muscle oil is applied and then get in the bath.

If stiffness continues in the morning, massage a small amount of the diluted mix into the area and repeat the bath.

Essential Oils That Help

Ginger	Camomile roman
Marjoram	Cardamom
Rosemary	Helichrysum

Other Care

It's important that in the case of overexercized muscles, only warmth is applied, because it increases the flow of blood to the area. Put a hot water bottle or hot pad against the overexercized muscle, or if the muscle is in a leg or arm, wrap it in warm towels.

When to Get Help

Get help if the pain is very severe, and the child can't lift the affected limb, or walk, easily.

Prevention

- Teach your child to stretch and do warm up exercises before and after doing any sports, dance, or other strenuous physical activity.

PIN WORM
(THREADWORMS — ENTEROBIUS VERMICULARIS)

This is a very common parasitic infection, usually found in children between the ages of 5 and 9. The worms are about 1 cm long and thin — resembling a piece of white cotton thread. They live in the child's intestines and usually come out at night, often causing the child to wake up and complain of itching around the anal or vulva area.

The eggs can easily be passed from person to person. Although the eggs can be breathed in through the air, the most usual way for a child to become infected is by handling contaminated objects such as toys, clothing, even furniture and toilet seats, and then putting their fingers in their mouths. It's important to wipe down all areas that may have eggs left on them.

Essential oils can be used as a complementary treatment to the medication available through your doctor or drug store. The American Medical Association recommends baths to soothe the anal area.

Signs and Symptoms

- itching around buttocks or anus, and sometimes vagina — especially shortly after going to bed
- disturbed sleep
- red, irritated skin around anus
- white, thread-like worms in stools
- irritability, seems generally unwell
- pin worms and other parasites may be responsible for: weight loss, swollen abdomen, inability to concentrate, lethargy, headaches, teeth-grinding, and dribbling saliva during night

Tummy Massage	*Soothing Lotion*	*Baths*
Into one ounce sesame seed oil, mix the following: *3 drops clove* *6 drops niaouli* *10 drops cardamom* *8 drops bay* *Rub a small amount of the mix over the child's back and stomach area. Cover with a warm, dry compress until cool. Then massage a small amount of plain sesame oil over the stomach only. Use for no longer than one week.*	*To help soothe the area, bathe the anus with a small amount of the following:* *First mix together:* *¹/₂ ounce aloe vera gel* *¹/₂ ounce camomile water* *¹/₂ ounce lavender water* *Then add:* *2 drops lavender* *1 drop cardamom* *Mix well, and soothe a small amount around the anus after using the bathroom.*	*In one teaspoon vegetable oil mix the following:* *4 drops cardamom* *3 drops camomile roman* *Use ¹/₄ teaspoon in a bath for children between 5 and 7 years, and ¹/₂ teaspoon for older children.*

Essential Oils That Help

Niaouli	Fennel
Lavender	Cardamom
Camomile roman	Clove
Bay	

Other Care

Use medications available from your doctor or drug store. Give the child plenty of cabbage, onions, and garlic, and have them drink pomegranate juice frequently.

Herbal tinctures such as black walnut are available in health stores. The worms come out of the body to lay their eggs. To encourage the worms to come out of the body have the child sit in a bowl of warm milk. The worms are attracted by the warm milk. If the child can be made to pass feces at this time, all the better. Do this after medication has been taken. Read to the child to distract them from what is happening. Afterward, wash the child's bottom in soap and warm water.

Prevention

- Teach children to wash their hands thoroughly with soap after going to the bathroom, and before snacks and mealtimes.
- Put a couple drops of essential oil on tissues and wipe over toilet seats.
- When using public bathrooms, teach girls to pass urine while slightly standing so they don't touch the toilet seat.
- In the household, use the spray method to put a fine mist of essential oils in the air to discourage airborne eggs.

PNEUMONIA

Pneumonia attacks the lungs. The infection can be caused by a virus, bacteria, or fungus. There are two types: the first type affects the air passages and then spreads to the lungs; the second type affects the lobes of the lungs. One or both lungs can be infected.

Pneumonia can be caught by breathing in infected air. It can also develop from bacteria which are normally present in the nose and throat of the infected person, especially when their resistance to disease is low. As the symptoms are so like those of many other diseases, it can be difficult for a parent to decide if the child has the infection or not. It can start with cold-like symptoms, often with a cough. The treatment of pneumonia with pharmacological antibiotics has been very good.

Signs and Symptoms

- can start with cold-like symptoms: cough, stuffed up nose, tiredness
- high temperature or fever, yet child may feel chilly
- difficulty in breathing, may wheeze
- chest pains, lung ache or pain
- produces phlegm
- headache
- abdominal pains
- lips and nails look bluish

Bed Socks

Put the following essential oils on the inside sole of two bedsocks:

1 drop thyme linalol
1 drop ginger

Put the socks on your child's feet, and keep the feet warm.

Pneumonia Mix

The following mix can be used in several ways. Follow the directions in the boxes below. First mix the following:

10 drops ravensara
10 drops eucalyptus citriodora
5 drops niaouli
5 drops thyme linalol

Body Rub

A massage over the back and upper chest can make breathing less difficult.

Use a small amount of the following mix each time:

$^{1}/_{2}$ ounce vegetable oil
10 drops pneumonia mix above

Baths

Dilute 3 drops of the pneumonia mix in $^{1}/_{2}$ teaspoon vegetable oil. If your child is 7 years of age or over, use the entire amount. If your child is 6 or under, use half this amount. Add to the bath water, and swish around well before your child gets in.

Diffuser

In one of the room methods use:

5 drops pneumonia mix above
5 drops cinnamon

If you use a diffuser, do not leave it in your child's room overnight.

Tissue or Pillow

Put 1–2 drops pneumonia mix on a tissue for the child to sniff when needed.

Put 1–2 drops pneumonia mix on pillows, under the corner, away from the eyes.

Fevers

Sponge Method

This method is particularly helpful if your child is hot and sticky.

Prepare a bowl of luke-warm, not cold, water, to which you've added 2 drops lavender. Soak a sponge, squeeze it out, and use to wipe down your child's body.

Vinegar Method

This method has been a favorite with Europeans for generations.

Prepare with the following:

1 bowl of luke-warm water
2 tablespoons vinegar
3 drops lavender

Put a piece of cloth or plain, unprinted brown paper in the bowl, squeeze out, then place it over the forehead of the child, making sure nothing drips into the eyes. When it heats up, remove it, and repeat the procedure.

Compress and Massage

Sleep is important. The following method may help your child sleep.

Add the following essential oils to a bowl of cool, but not cold, water:

1 drop camomile roman
1 drop lavender
1 drop lemon
1 drop coriander

Dip a compress in the water and squeeze out. Place over your child's back for about 5 minutes. Make sure the water isn't cold, but pleasantly cool to the child. Then dry the skin, and massage the back with this oil:

1 teaspoon vegetable oil
2 drops rose otto
1 drop lavender

If your child has a fever, try one of the remedies below to bring the temperature down.

Essential Oils That Help

Ravensara	Tea tree
Niaouli	Thyme linalol
Elemi	

Other Care

Give your child plenty of liquids. They should rest, and if you prop the child up in bed that will ease the coughing and make breathing easier. Open the windows so fresh air can circulate freely.

When to Get Help

Contact your doctor immediately if your child has any of the symptoms listed above, and you believe your child may have contracted pneumonia. Once diagnosed, get additional medical help as soon as possible if your child experiences any difficulty in breathing.

Prevention

Prevention is directed at trying to ensure other members of the family do not contract pneumonia. Elderly people and babies are especially at risk.

- Keep other members of the household away from the child with pneumonia.
- Other members of the household could use 4 drops of the pneumonia mix of essential oils in the bath.
- Diffuse antiviral essential oils throughout the home or Antiinfectious Air Spray on page 37

POISON IVY

See also: Hives

Poison ivy is one of the three main poisonous plants in the U.S. The other two are poison oak and poison sumac. Contact with poison ivy causes a severe skin reaction. The plant has three shiny green leaves attached to a single stem, which turn red in the fall. It's the oil in the sap that causes the rash, and a child can be affected from anything the sap has been in direct contact with — even the fur on a pet. Symptoms appear 1 to 4 days after being in contact with the sap. It's not contagious, and will heal itself within 2 to 3 weeks if left alone. However, it's very itchy and sore, and can be painful.

Signs and Symptoms

- an itchy, blistering red rash anywhere on the body; can be in patches or lines
- blisters often weep a fluid
- the area is swollen

The oat bath and calamine lotion methods are helpful in cases of poison ivy. Follow the instructions for these in Chickenpox, Eczema, or Hives. In all cases, first wash the affected area thoroughly with soap and water.

Cold Compress	Cool Showers
Use a cool compress to help soothe the rash. Add the following essential oils to a small bowl of water:	*A cool shower will help relieve the itching. Put the following essential oils onto a wet wash cloth:*
4 drops camomile german *2 drops helichrysum* *4 drops lavender*	*2 drops camomile roman* *2 drops camomile german*
Soak the compress in the water, squeeze out, and apply to the rash.	*Gently apply the wash cloth over the affected area.*

Essential Oils That Help

Camomile german	Camomile roman
Lavender	Eucalyptus radiata
Helichrysum	

Other Care

Wash your child's clothes with a strong detergent; if you're camping, use the strongest soap you have with you. Keep the child from scratching as much as possible.

When to Get Help

Get help if you are not sure whether your child's rash is actually a reaction to poison ivy. If it is poison ivy, your child may be allergic to the plant and need medication, such as antihistamine. Get medical help if the rash covers a large part of your child's body; or seems to be infected. Also get medical help if your child has breathing difficulties, vomiting, headache, or is feeling dizzy; or if the rash spreads to your child's face, eyes, lips, or nose.

Prevention

- Have your child wear trousers and long sleeves in areas where poison ivy grows.
- Washing the area immediately after contact sometimes stops the rash from developing.

PSORIASIS

Psoriasis is a skin condition with dry, scaly patches, that can come on in childhood, or adulthood. The severity of the condition changes very much from person to person. There may be small patches that come up all over the body, or larger patches, for example on the elbows and knees. In really severe cases, a large part of the body's surface can be covered. There are different types of the condition; in children the most common type is a mild form called glutate psoriasis.

Why a person should develop psoriasis is unknown, but various triggers can cause outbreaks, including having an infection, an injury on the skin, or being under stress. The winter months can make it worse because the skin isn't being exposed to the sun. Psoriasis appears to run in families, and you often find that other members of the child's family have hay fever, or are asthmatic.

Signs and Symptoms
- can start with tiny bumps of reddish-pink flaky skin areas — behind the knees, in the crook of the elbow, lower back, on the scalp, or hair-line
- scales look silvery and flake off easily
- skin may crack and become painful — risk of infection
- joints can swell, become painful, or ache

All types of psoriasis are different, and a lot depends on the constitution of the particular child. There is no overall remedy that will be effective for all children.

Oat Baths

Oat baths can be wonderfully soothing to the skin. Use raw organic oats or oatmeal. Put a pile of oats or oatmeal onto a piece of material, and add the essential oils to them. Securely tie the bundle and attach it to the bath faucet, so the water runs through the oats before reaching the bath. There are 4 baths to choose from, as different children respond differently to particular oils:

Bath #1 add:	**Bath #2 add:**
4 drops camomile german	4 drops bergamot
Bath #3 add:	**Bath #4 add:**
1 drop spikenard	2 drops lavender

Oil Bath / Bicarbonate Bath

Oil Bath	**Bicarbonate Bath**
Use half of this mix in a bath:	*First add the following essential oils to 1 cup bicarbonate of soda:*
1 teaspoon almond oil	
1 drop lavender	
1 drop bergamot	2 drops lavender
1 drop geranium	1 drop camomile german
1 drop camomile roman	
Swish the water around well before your child gets in.	*Mix in well with a spoon, then add to the bath water. Swish the water around well before your child gets in.*

Skin Oil No. 1 / Skin Oil No. 2

Skin Oil No. 1	**Skin Oil No. 2**
Smooth a small amount over the patches of dry, flaky skin. Mix together well:	*Smooth a small amount over the patches of dry, flaky skin. Mix together well:*
1 ounce sesame seed oil	
1 ounce pure virgin olive oil	1 ounce calendula infused oil
Then add:	4 drops bergamot
	3 drops camomile roman
25 drops red carrot oil	
5 drops borage seed oil	
3 drops geranium	
And mix together well.	

Essential Oils That Help

Camomile german   Camomile roman
Lavender   Bergamot
Spikenard   Rose otto

Other Care

Certain foods make the condition worse. These are: dairy products, wheat products, additives, preservatives, food coloring, and manufactured foods. Sodas, condiments, packaged sauces, and other prepared foods, are likely to make the condition worse.

Much as it may seem a daunting task, the long-term future of your child's psoriasis may depend to some degree on totally adjusting their diet, and possibly that of the family. You may like to follow The Cave Man Eating Plan on page 40. Basically, if a food walked, swam, or flew, you can eat it. If it grows out of the ground, that's fine, and if it's raw, that's better. Cereals, flours, and condiments should be organic. The whole family will enjoy more home cooking, and they'll feel better for it. Cutting out certain additives may even improve behavior. Buying organic products can cost more, but you'll save on sodas and prepared foods — and you may actually end up getting more for your money. It's got to be worth trying for a month.

When to Get Help

If you suspect your child may be developing psoriasis, consult your physician. The general prescription is hydrocortisone, and if it becomes more of a problem, steroid creams. Tar creams or baths may also be recommended. In European hospitals, a popular treatment for severe cases is the ultraviolet light from sunbeds.

RASHES

See also: Rashes — Newborn

Skin rashes are caused by many things and are often a symptom of infection or disease. A rash may be a reaction of the body's immune system as it fights off an invader. A rash is also often an allergic reaction to something that has touched or bitten the skin, or is in the atmosphere, or has been eaten. Parasites can sometimes cause rashes, or it can result from a serious blood condition. There are so many possible causes of skin rash, it can be hard to identify the cause in every case.

If there is a rash on your child's body, you need to look for other symptoms or causes. Has the child got a temperature or fever, or other signs of illness? Has your child been playing in long grass, or near woods? Make a note of whether the rash is spreading. Blood poisoning — septicemia — causes a rash that does not fade temporarily when a clear glass is pressed against it (see Meningitis). This rash starts as a group of very tiny blood spots, but these rapidly get bigger when they resemble fresh bruises with bleeding under the skin. If your child's rash is of this type, do not wait for medical help to come to you, take the child immediately to the nearest medical facility, and insist on being seen right away.

Rashes come in all shapes and sizes, and anywhere on the body. Some may be raised or bumpy, others are flat. Some are more like blisters; with others, the surrounding tissue may be swollen. The rash might be pink, red, or purple. The rash might be a series of spots joined together, or a continuous area of similarly disturbed skin. Some rashes are distinctive, and indicate a particular cause; while others could be caused by a variety of things. To help you identify the cause of your child's rash, refer to the Signs and Symptoms list in the individual sections.

Signs and Symptoms

- *rashes caused by a virus:* chickenpox, rubella — German measles, fifth disease, or hand, foot, and mouth disease
- *rashes caused by a bacteria:* meningitis, impetigo, scarlet fever
- *rashes caused by a fungus:* ringworm, thrush
- *rashes caused by a parasite:* scabies
- *rashes caused by an allergic reaction:* hives, contact dermatitis
- *rashes caused by an allergic reaction to:* poison ivy, poison oak, poison sumbac, other plants, chemicals, medications; foods such as strawberries, cherries, and eggs
- *rashes caused by an insect bite from:* bees, wasps, fleas, ants, mosquitoes
- *newborns:* thema toxicum, cradle cap, prickly heat (See Rashes — Newborns)

Baths

If your child has a rash, keep the skin cool, and give your child soothing baths. Add the following to a bath of tepid to warm water:

1 tablespoon bicarbonate of soda
1 tablespoon baking soda
2 drops camomile german
2 drops lavender

Essential Oils That Help

Camomile german	Lavender
Camomile roman	Helichrysum
Niaouli	Eucalyptus radiata

Other Care

Try to stop your child from scratching the rash, as this might lead to infection.

When to Get Help

Get medical help if your child has a temperature or fever. Also seek medical attention if the rash gets worse and spreads; if the rash is infected with pus; or is bleeding; or if it does not improve within 48 hours.

RASHES — NEWBORN

Figures show that 50 percent of newborn babies have rashes; certainly it is very common. The cause is not really known but a rash could just be the baby's skin getting acclimated to being out of the womb, or a reaction to the air on the skin, or a reaction to clothing. It's always worrisome when a newborn has a rash, especially for a first-time parent, so do get reassurance from your pediatrician.

Signs and Symptoms

- slightly raised red rash, on any part of body
- sometimes with a few pimples
- lasts 7 to 14 days

I prefer not to use essential oils on newborn babies, whose bodies are just getting used to a strange environment. If your newborn's skin is very dry, use a small amount of pure, virgin, organic olive oil and smooth it onto your baby's skin. Try to avoid baby oils, creams, and lotions, many of which contain petroleum by-products. The following two methods can safely be used on newborns if you follow the directions exactly. In warm weather, try to leave baby's skin exposed to the air as much as possible, rather than covering it in wool or other warm clothing.

Body Oil

This oil is effective in clearing up a newborn skin rash. Very little essential oil is used in the following mix, and you will only need to use a tiny amount each time. First mix the following:

1 ounce virgin, organic olive oil
1 drop camomile german

Put a tiny amount of the oil in the palm of one hand and rub both hands together. This spreads the oil so you don't use too much and helps to make the oil warm and comfortable to the baby. Then smooth your hands over the affected areas of the baby's skin. Do not leave baby's skin greasy; dab excess off with a soft piece of material.

Hydrolat/Water Lotion

See page 12 for how to make an essential oil "water." First combine the following:

$1/4$ ounce lavender hydrolat (or "water")
$1/4$ ounce camomile (or "water")

Take half this amount, and add to $1/4$ ounce warm (not hot) pure bottled water.
Add a few grains of salt. Use a small sponge to dab gently on baby's rash. Pat dry.

Essential Oils That Help

Camomile german

When to Get Help

Consult your pediatrician if you are unsure what the rash is, or if it doesn't clear up in 14 hours. If any children in the home or neighborhood have a contagious infection of any kind, get medical advice.

RINGWORM

Strictly speaking, ringworm refers to a large group of different fungal infections. What people generally know as ringworm is a skin infection that looks a bit like a bull's eye, circular or ring-shaped, with an unaffected area in the middle. The outer ring of ringworm marks the active area of the fungus. The center heals as the fungus moves outwards, making the circle larger.

Ringworm is caused by a highly contagious fungus called tinea, and can spread quickly around a school. It's caught by contact with the fungus, either directly by touching infected skin, or indirectly by sharing the belongings of an infected person, such as clothes, hats, brushes, combs, towels, washcloths, or pillows. It's most common in children between the ages of 2 and 10, and can last up to six weeks.

Signs and Symptoms

- a reddish-pink, circular, slightly raised mark on the skin — the center is unaffected
- found anywhere on the body, but particularly: the face, limbs, groin, and scalp — where it can cause patches of hair loss
- the patches can enlarge and the area can become itchy with scaly skin
- sometimes pus-filled lumpy swellings
- due to the child scratching the ringworm: fingernails may be infected — pitted, thick, and discolored

Ringworm Mix

This can be used in the two methods below. Follow the instructions in the boxes.

First mix the following essential oils:

5 drops tea tree
5 drops manuka
8 drops neem oil

Neat	Evening Body Oil
Use 1 drop ringworm mix directly over the infected area. Do this 3 times a day.	*Dilute 3 drops ringworm mix in 1 teaspoon sesame oil. In the evening use it to rub over the whole body, avoiding the genital area. If the ringworm is very itchy, use over the affected area during the day as well.*

Shower Method

A warm shower will help to ease the itchy skin. Directly after the shower, while your child is still standing in the shower cubicle, gently pour camomile hydrolat/"water" over your child's body. See pages 11–12 for how to prepare essential oil hydrolats or "waters."

Scalp Treatment

Mix the following essential oils:

10 drops manuka (or kanuka)
20 drops neem
20 drops tea tree
10 drops palmarosa
10 drops geranium

Put 20 drops of the scalp treatment mix in 3 ounces plain, antiallergen, mild, baby shampoo and mix well. Use enough to shampoo the hair, and rinse well with water.

Then dilute 4 drops of the scalp treatment mix above in 1 tablespoon sesame oil, and apply all over the scalp — making sure none reaches the eyes, ears, nose, or mouth. Leave it in place for 10 minutes. Wash the hair again, using plain shampoo.

As a final rinse water, use 2 ounces of water to which you have added 3 drops of the essential oil mix above. Pour it over the scalp and hair, making sure to avoid the eyes, ears, nose, and mouth. Treat all the family with the same method, whether they're infected or not.

Essential Oils That Help

Lavender   Tea tree
Manuka   Neem
Palmarosa   Geranium

When to Get Help

Get medical advice if you are uncertain that your child's skin condition is ringworm. Also, get help if the ringworm is on the face or scalp; if it seems to be infected; or if it doesn't clear up after two weeks of any form of treatment.

Prevention

- Prevention consists of trying to stop the spread of infection.
- Cover the area with a dressing.
- Make sure the affected child's washcloth, towel, pillows, and clothes are not shared.
- Try to stop the affected child having close contact with other children and family members until the infection has cleared up.

ROCKY MOUNTAIN SPOTTED FEVER

Rocky mountain spotted fever is an infection caused by a bacteria called *rickettsia*, that is spread through the bite of a tic that lives in woods, or on dogs. It is a serious condition that requires immediate medical attention as soon as possible. The symptoms may not appear until 7 to 10 days after being bitten; it is not contagious.

Signs and Symptoms

- often starts with flu-like symptoms: high temperature or fever, chills, muscular aches and pains, severe headache
- a rash of small red spots that changes into a bruise-like area
- the rash starts on the wrists, palms of the hands, soles of the feet, and ankles, before spreading over the rest of the body
- can cause: stiff neck, red eyes, vomiting, confusion, seizures

Rocky mountain spotted fever is a very serious condition that requires proper diagnosis and medical treatment. Home help can be carried out alongside this to help ease the symptoms.

Rocky Mountain Spotted Fever (RMSF) Mix

The following mix can be used in several different ways. Follow the instructions in the boxes below.

Mix together the following essential oils:

20 drops thyme linalol
15 drops lavender
30 drops niaouli
10 drops helichrysum

Cool Baths	**Sponging**
Use 3 drops of the RMSF mix in cool baths.	If your child has a fever, sponge them down with tepid water. Add 6 drops of the RMSF mix to a small bowl of water.
Body Oil	**Diffusers**
Dilute 4 drops of the RMSF mix in 1 teaspoon vegetable oil. Gently rub it onto your child's body, avoiding the genital area.	Use 8 drops of the RMSF mix in a diffuser or other room method. Put the diffuser in your child's room, but do not leave it there overnight.

Essential Oils That Help

Thyme linalol	Lavender
Camomile german	Ravensara
Niaouli	Tea tree

Other Care

Give your child plenty of fluid to drink. Bed rest is essential. Try to keep your child cool, in a room that is warm, but has fresh air.

When to Get Help

Get immediate medical attention if your child is bitten by a tic whether you are able to remove the tic or not. Consult your physician as soon as any of the above symptoms appear, especially the rash.

Prevention

- If in wooded areas where these tics may live, put your child in a hat, a long sleeved top, and trousers that can be tucked into socks.
- Use insect repellents. See Lyme Disease for an effective deterrent clothing spray.

RUBELLA — GERMAN MEASLES

Rubella is a milder form of measles. It's inconvenient, but not harmful — unless it's caught by a woman during the first four months of pregnancy, when it can cause serious defects to the unborn child. If a female has not had German measles during her childhood, she can be vaccinated against it when she's a young woman so that if she comes into contact with rubella when she later becomes pregnant, it doesn't cause her any problems. The most important thing to remember, if your child has rubella, is to keep them out of contact with pregnant women until the infection has passed.

Rubella is a viral infection that causes a rash — that may start with just a small patch, usually behind the ears, but can spread and cover almost the whole body. It lasts anywhere from 3 to 15 days. Other symptoms may include mild fever and swollen glands. It's sometimes difficult to tell from the symptoms whether a child has rubella, or another type of rash or infection.

Rubella is an airborne infection that seems to be most active during the spring months. It's spread by an infected person sneezing or coughing, and the infected air being breathed in. The incubation time is generally 14 to 21 days although the rash can appear as early as three days after the virus has been contracted. A child is infectious during the time they have the rash, and for up to seven days after it has disappeared. Most children are immunized against this disease, but some still contract rubella even after immunization.

Signs and Symptoms
- runny nose, other cold-like symptoms
- a small rash appears — usually starts behind the ears, then spreads to the body
- can be: mild fever; glands behind the ears are swollen

When a child has rubella, rest and plenty of fluid are the order of the day. Use an antiviral mix of essential oil in the diffuser or spray methods to help stop the spread of the virus to other members of the household. The spots in the rash can be very itchy, and soothing baths help stop the irritation. Use warm, not hot, water in baths.

Aloe Vera Bath	To Help Sleep Bath
Use 4 drops of the essential oil mix (below) added to 1 ounce aloe vera water and 1 ounce lavender "water." Add the entire mix to the bath water:	The following combination of essential oils will not only soothe the rash, but help the child get a good night's sleep.
5 drops lavender 3 drops camomile roman 3 drops camomile german 4 drops bergamot	Put the following essential oils in 1 teaspoon vegetable oil, then add to the bath water. Swish around well before the child gets in.
Use 4 drops only. Swish the water around well before the child gets in.	2 drops geranium 2 drops lavender 1 drops petitgrain

Swollen Glands

Use about a dime-size amount of this oil. Apply gently over the glands behind both ears, and down the neck and into the armpits:

1 tablespoon vegetable oil
10 drops thyme linalol

Essential Oils That Help

Lavender
Camomile roman
Geranium
Ravensara

Thyme linalol
Tea tree
Bergamot

Other Care

Keep your child away from pregnant women, and other members of the family. Put your child to bed only if they are feeling unwell.

When to Get Help

Always inform your doctor if your child catches rubella. If your child complains of a stiff neck, or if their temperature rises, consult your doctor again.

Prevention

- Immunization is available.
- To help prevent the infection spreading to other people, use antiviral essential oils around the home — in the diffuser and spray methods.

SHOCK

Shock often follows after an injury, blood loss, pain, fear, bereavement, or an emotional trauma such as seeing an accident or violent incident. The shock can come on immediately, or very slowly. Shock is very dangerous and can cause physical damage if not treated medically. There are many circumstances in which shock may occur, and whenever there has been physical damage to a child, or another person within their sight, or emotional trauma, the symptoms should be looked for, bearing in mind that shock may occur some time after the shocking event.

Signs and Symptoms

- child feels cold
- clammy skin
- blood appears to drain from the face, which can become very pale
- dry mouth
- breathing quickens; breathing becomes shallow; hyperventilation
- pulse can quicken; or become faint
- unable to move — frozen and trance-like
- child carries on but with slow, mechanical movements, little reaction, and staring eyes

---

Inhalation

Since mankind first noticed the power of smell, essential oils and other fragrant materials have been given to people in shock as a treatment. Smelling salts are not appropriate in cases of shock.

Use 1 drop of any of the following essential oils. Put the essential oil onto a tissue or piece of cloth and pass it under the child's nose. In an emergency, just pass the essential oil bottle under the child's nose. Use any of the following:

camomile roman
geranium
lemon

Comforting Hand or Foot Massage

A child often needs comforting after having mild shock which requires no medication or hospital treatment. This may be the case if the child has had a scary experience. A light, comforting massage of the hands or feet, or both, can work wonders, especially when combined with cuddles.

Use the following mix:

1 teaspoon vegetable oil
1 drop mandarin (or tangerine)
1 drop petitgrain

Essential Oils That Help

Lemon	Geranium
Camomile roman	Rose

Other Care

If an injury has occurred, do not move your child. If no neck, back, or head injury has occurred, raise their head slightly, but not their legs. If there has been no injury to the child, lie them down, and raise their legs above their head, to encourage the flow of blood to the heart and brain. Cover your child with whatever is available to keep them warm.

There are certain prepared natural remedies for shock: Dr. Bach's "Rescue Remedy" or "Five Flower Essence Healing Herbs," homeopathic arnica tablets, "Front Line" Mother Essences.

When to Get Help

If your child is in shock, they need immediate emergency medical attention.

Prevention

If a disaster has occurred:

- Cover your child.
- Comfort your child by rubbing their hands.

SINUSITIS

Sinusitis is an inflammation of the lining of the sinuses. There are many causes, including hay fever, allergy, nasal injury, being in a smoky atmosphere, ear problems, or infections of the throat, teeth, or gums, colds, and flu.

Signs and Symptoms

- nasal congestion
- headache
- sore and swollen eyes, can feel as if they are throbbing
- pain around the cheek bones and forehead
- fatigue, feeling generally unwell
- in serious cases there can be: a thick yellow/greenish nasal discharge

Steam Methods

Steam often helps the child breathe more easily, and essential oils can be added in the following methods.

Bowl Method	Inhalation	Bathrooms
Put a bowl of steaming water in the child's room, and add the following essential oils: 4 drops ravensara 4 drops niaouli 4 drops camomile roman Ensure the bowl is out of reach of children and pets.	An older child can use the inhalation method. Make up the mix of essential oils to the left, and use 4 drops in a bowl of steaming water. The child should inhale this, leaning over the bowl with their head covered, mouth and eyes closed. Menthol crystals — available from drug stores — can also be used in this inhalation.	If the sinuses are really bad and your child can find no relief, the very steamy atmosphere of a bathroom may help. The child should not get in the bath. Run a very hot bath, and keep the door closed. Have the child sit in the bathroom — not in the bath — and inhale the steam through their nose. Add the complete sinusitis mix, on page 242, to the water — this is many drops, but remember that nobody is getting in the bath.

Compresses

Compresses can help relieve the congestion. You can use either warm or hot compresses, depending on which your child finds more effective at the time.

First add the following essential oils to a bowl containing 1 pint of warm or hot water:

4 drops rosemary
2 drops eucalyptus radiata
6 drops ravensara

Place a compress or wash cloth in the water, squeeze it out well, and place over your child's forehead. Make sure no water goes into their eyes. An older child can hold the compress in place. As the compress starts to dry, have another ready to use. You should get at least 4 compresses out of one bowl of water.

Sinusitis Mix

The following mix of essential oils can be used in the methods below. Follow the instructions in each box.

First mix the following essential oils together:

6 drops ravensara
5 drops niaouli
2 drops eucalyptus radiata
4 drops camomile roman

Forehead Oil	Tissue	Pillow
Put a tiny amount of the following mix on one fingertip and smooth it over the forehead and nose, being careful to avoid the eye area: *1 teaspoon vegetable oil* *3 drops of the sinusitis mix* *1 drop camomile german* *With a tissue, gently dab off any excess oil which has not soaked into the skin.*	*Put 1 drop of the sinusitis mix on a tissue.* *Give it to your child to inhale during the day.*	*At night, put 1 drop of the sinusitis mix on your child's pillow — under a corner, away from the eyes.* *Use extra pillows to prop your child up higher.*

Essential Oils That Help

Ravensara   Niaouli
Tea tree   Camomile roman
Eucalyptus radiata   Rosemary

Other Care

Salt water nose drops are often used, and are available at drug stores. A hot, dry, stuffy atmosphere makes the condition worse, so keep your child's room aired, and use a humidifier or similar method to keep the air moist overnight. Give your child plenty of fluids to drink, including fruit juices, and avoid dairy products for a while as these can cause more mucus in the body.

When to Get Help

Get medical help if the headache turns into a throb; if the condition lasts for longer than three days; or if there is a thick yellow/greenish nasal discharge that lasts longer than three days.

SORE THROAT — STREP THROAT

Children often complain of sore throats, which more often than not are gone by the next morning. The throat irritation is usually caused by a bacteria or virus. "Strep" throat is caused by the streptococcus bacteria, and usually clears up within a few days. However, a sore throat can be a symptom of a more serious condition, and certain steps need to be taken to decide if this is the case.

Take your child's temperature, and check whether their glands are swollen. Ask if they have difficulty swallowing. Use a spoon to hold down your child's tongue, and check to see if there is any inflammation, redness, or swelling, of the throat or tonsils. Look to see if there are any white spots. A sore throat could be a symptom of several conditions including cold, flu, laryngitis, mumps, nephritis, rheumatic fever, scarlet fever, and tonsillitis, and may require medical advice. The following suggestions can be used quite safely with any medication.

Signs and Symptoms

- pain in the throat
- difficulty in swallowing
- swollen lymph glands
- red and swollen tonsils
- white spots on the tonsils

Sore Throat Drink

Drinks can help ease the soreness in the throat. The following soothing drink can be given to children over 3 years of age. If your child is younger, omit the lemon essential oil.

First mix together well:

4 ounces hot water
1 teaspoon runny honey
2 tablespoons cooking rose water
the juice of 1 lemon
1 drop lemon essential oil

Then pour the mixture through an unbleached paper coffee filter. When the drink is cool, give it to your child to sip. Cover the drink, and leave it by your child's side, so they can sip it when they feel the need. Very young children can be given the drink by spoon.

Throat Oil

Use a small amount of the following oil to rub over the throat area. First mix together the following essential oils:

4 drops tea tree
2 drops lemon
5 drops ravensara
4 drops thyme linalol
5 drops manuka (or additional tea tree)

Dilute 5 drops of the mix in 1 teaspoon vegetable oil. This will be enough for several applications.

Swollen Glands Oil

Thyme linalol or manuka essential oil can be used in high dosage over the glands on either side of the neck. Put 1 drop of your chosen essential oil on a fingertip, plus 1 drop vegetable oil. Rub your fingertips together, and smooth over the glands.

Essential Oils That Help

Tea tree	Camomile roman
Thyme linalol	Ravensara
Helichrysum	Manuka
Ginger	Eucalyptus radiata
Cajeput	Geranium

Other Care

See the advice in Laryngitis. Keep your child away from school. Give them plenty to drink, and liquify all foods. To soothe the throat, give your child ice cream and frozen fruit juice popsicles. If the throat is inflamed, warm compresses applied to the throat sometimes help.

When to Get Help

Consult your physician if there are white spots anywhere in the mouth or throat; if your child has a temperature or fever, a rash, a headache, or aches and pains.

SPLINTERS

A splinter is a small foreign object embedded in the skin or flesh. Most splinters that a child is likely to get will be from wood, thorns, or plastic. Rarely is metal involved, unless the child spends time in garages or workshops where metal shavings are present. Most splinters can easily be removed at home.

Signs and Symptoms
- small object visible beneath skin
- pain, soreness
- can become infected if not removed

If the splinter is visible and can be firmly grasped, remove it very carefully with a pair of tweezers. The whole splinter must be removed to avoid the risk of infection. If the splinter is caught in the skin, softening the area with warm water before trying to remove the splinter may help. But don't try this if the splinter is made of wood, as soaking will just make the wood soft and more likely to break, and it will become impossible to remove it easily. After removing the splinter, wash the area well with soap and water, and apply 1 drop of one of the following essential oils.

Essential Oils That Help

Myrrh	Thyme linalol
Tea tree	Manuka

Other Care

Use disinfectant or tea tree in the washing water. If the hole in the skin is large enough to require covering with a Band-Aid, keep an eye on it to make sure no infection develops.

When to Get Help

Get help if the splinter is too deeply embedded into the skin to allow removal, or if the end of the splinter breaks off into the skin, so you can't remove it. In the days following the removal of a splinter, look for signs of infection, such as reddening of the tissue, or a whitish-yellow area under the skin, that could indicate pus developing.

Prevention

- Use sandpaper to smooth rough edges of wooden furniture, fences, door frames, etc.
- Keep children away from areas where metal or plastic cutting or shaving is taking place, or has taken place.
- Survey your home to check there are no objects or furniture which might give your child a splinter.

SPRAINS — LIGAMENTS

See also: Strains — Pulled Muscles

A sprain is what happens when a ligament tears, or gets over-stretched. A ligament is the fibrous tissue that holds the bones of a joint together. Gymnasts and dancers are very prone to this injury, as are energetic and sporty children. The most usual place children get a sprain is in an ankle, as they make a sudden twist, or slip sideways in their shoe. Sprains are caused by any type of pulling or wrenching movement. Sprains are graded in terms of severity on a scale of 1 to 3, with 3 being the most serious.

Signs and Symptoms

- mostly affects ankles, knees, wrists, shoulders, elbows
- pain and swelling in the area
- difficulty moving the area without increased pain
- tenderness when touched
- stiffness, cramps, bruising
- third grade sprains: if the ligament has completely torn away from the bone, the joint can't hold the bones in place and the joint will be very wobbly
- if there is a tear, but the ligament is still attached, it will be very painful, but the joint will still be stable

After a sprain, the area should be rested. If the sprain is in the ankle or knee, raise your child's leg. This will help reduce the flow of blood to the area, and prevent further swelling. Apply an icepack to the area, or bathe with iced water to help reduce the swelling.

Cold Compresses

Cold compresses will help to reduce the swelling.

Add the following essential oils to a bowl of water:

lavender
camomile roman

Put the compress in the water, squeeze it out, and apply to the area of the sprain.

Sprain (and Strain) Oil

For minor sprains, prepare the following mix:

1 dessertspoon vegetable oil
4 drops black pepper
3 drops ginger
4 drops helichrysum

Smooth a small amount of the oil onto the affected area.

Over–8 Sprain (and Strain) Oil

The following oil can be used on children over 8 years of age.

First blend the following:

20 drops helichrysum
20 drops vegetable oil

Use between 2–6 drops of this oil, depending on the size of the affected area. Put the oil directly on the sprain, three times a day, for 2 days only.

Essential Oils That Help

Ginger	Thyme linalol
Lavender	Camomile roman
Eucalyptus radiata	Ormenis flower (Camomile Maroc)
Helichrysum	Black pepper

Other Care

Apply the physical and sports therapist's R.I.C.E. rule: rest, ice, compression, elevation. *Rest:* There should be no exercise until the area has healed. *Ice:* Crush ice in a plastic bag, wrap in a towel, and apply to the area. Alternatively, freeze water in a polystyrene cup and, when it's frozen, cut the sides down slightly so there's a block you can apply directly onto the injured area. Apply the ice method for a few minutes, take the ice away for 5 minutes, then apply again. *Compression:* Wrap the area in an elastic bandage, making sure it supports the area, but is not so tight the area can't be moved, or circulation is restricted. In the case of a shoulder, elbow, or wrist, use a sling to restrict movement, and prevent further damage. *Elevation:* If the injury is in the ankle or knee, raise the injured area so it's higher than the heart.

When to Get Help

Get help if you suspect a fracture; if the bone looks out of shape or bent; or if the joint is wobbly. Also get help if your child is in a great deal of pain, even when the area is not being moved; or if after two days the area is more swollen, and painful to the touch.

Prevention

- Put your child in shoes that properly support the feet.
- If your child is sporty, ensure they wear shoes that are designed for the particular sport they partake in.
- Ensure that the sports equipment your child is using is of the correct size and weight for their body weight.

STRAINS — PULLED MUSCLES

See also: Overexercised Muscles

A strain refers to a tear or over-stretching of the muscular fibers or tendons. Strained muscles can occur anywhere in the body and are very painful. However, most strains are minor and will respond to home treatment and rest fairly quickly. The treatment for strains is similar, in some respects, to that for sprains — which is why in this section you will find similar information, and some references to the Sprains section.

Signs and Symptoms

- pain and soreness in the muscle, hurts to move the area
- can affect anywhere — stomach, limbs, neck et cetera.

Rest the strained area completely. If the strain is in the leg or arm, raise that limb to help reduce blood flow, and reduce swelling in the area. Apply an icepack to the area, or bathe with iced water.

Cold Compress

Follow the instructions for the Cold Compress method in Sprains. (See page 208.)

Strain Oil No. 1

First mix the following essential oils together:

5 drops ginger
2 drops black pepper
5 drops marjoram
5 drops ormenis flower (camomile maroc)
5 drops helichrysum

Dilute a number of drops of this essential oil mix in 1 teaspoon vegetable oil. How many drops you need to use will depend on the age of your child — see page 24 for the general rule guidelines. When diluted, smooth the oil over the injured area. Then bandage the area, if the location of the strain makes that possible.

Strain Oil No. 2

Follow the instructions for the Sprain (and Strain) Oil in Sprains (see page 209).

Over 8 Strain Oil

Follow the instructions for the Over-8 Sprain (and Strain) Oil in Sprains (see page 209).

Essential Oils That Help

Ginger	Thyme linalol
Lavender	Camomile roman
Eucalyptus radiata	Ormenis flower (Camomile Maroc)
Helichrysum	Black pepper

Other Care

If the strain is in a muscle in an arm or leg, bandage the area to give support, making sure it's not too tight. Don't let your child exercise until the strained area has healed. Your child may benefit from the following natural remedies: Dr Bach's Rescue Remedy, Five Flower Essence Healing Herbs, homeopathic arnica tablets, or Front Line Mother Essences.

When to Get Help

Get immediate medical help if your child experiences pain in an area of the body other than the area of the strain. Also, get help if your child is in severe pain that does not ease; or if swelling or inflammation develop. If, after 48 hours of resting, the strain does not appear to be improving, get medical advice.

Prevention

- As all dancers and athletes know, you should always stretch before exercising, and keep the muscles warm during and after exercise. Teach your child this important information.
- Also teach your child not to push their body to achieve too much too soon — going at the right pace is important.

STY

A sty is a bacterial infection that causes an inflamed, pus-filled sac on the edge of the upper or lower eye lid. It's often situated near the eyelashes. The sty can appear rather like a small boil, causing redness and swelling of the eye lid, which can make the eye seem almost closed. Sties can spread to other areas of the same eye, or from eye to eye, so hygiene is very important.

Signs and Symptoms

- itchiness, soreness, redness, and swelling of the eye lid
- becomes a lump under the skin, eventually turning into a pimple-type head of yellow pus

Do not attempt to squeeze out the pus or remove it in any way — the body must be left to deal with the sty as best it can. Warm, wet compresses can give some relief, and help to soften the lump area, possibly bringing out the pus.

Hydrolat-Water Compress

First turn to page 11 and read the section on hydrolats, so you are very clear about what these are. Boil the following together:

1 tablespoon lavender hydrolat
1 tablespoon camomile hydrolat
2 tablespoons pure spring water
1 teaspoon witch hazel

Allow to cool down. When the mix is still slightly warm, put a small piece of muslin or similar light material in it. Squeeze out the excess liquid and lay the muslin over the closed eye. Do this at least 4 times a day.

You can use the hyrolat-water mix above also to simply dab on the area of the sty — but only if you can avoid getting the mix into the eye itself. The child must be old enough to understand they must keep their eye tightly shut. Don't use cotton wool to dab the area because little bits may get into the eye, and irritate it more.

Filter Method of Compress

First turn to page 11 and read the section on hydrolats and "waters," so you are very clear about what these are.

1 tablespoon rose water
1 tablespoon camomile hydrolat/"water"
1 drop camomile roman
2 tablespoons pure spring water
1 teaspoon witch hazel

Heat the above ingredients, then pour through an unbleached paper coffee filter. Do not forget the paper filter part of these instructions.

When cooled, use in the compress method: dipping muslin in the liquid mix, squeezing it out well, and applying over the sty area. The eye must be tightly closed, so this can only be used with children who can be trusted to do that.

You can use the mix above also to simply dab on the area of the sty — but only if you can avoid getting it into the eye itself. Don't use cotton balls for this application.

Cheek Oil

This oil is for putting on the cheek bone. Do not put it anywhere around the eye at all. Apply very little — just a dab. Wipe off any excess with a tissue right away.

Mix together:

$^1/_2$ teaspoon vegetable oil
lavender – 5 drops

Apply only a tiny amount with a fingertip along the cheek bone.

Essential Oils That Help

You cannot use any essential oils in the eye area. However, thoroughly sterilized essential oil hydrolats or "waters" can be used in the compress or lid-bathing methods.

Other Care

The sty will disappear without any help, around 5 days after the pus has gone. Unfortunately, new ones often appear, close to the original site. Some children are very prone to sties, and good nutrition is important to them.

When to Get Help

Get medical advice if the redness and swelling carry on for a long time; if the sty seems to be getting worse, or doesn't seem to be disappearing; if there are a cluster of sties; or if the sty is still there after two weeks.

SUNBURN

See also: Heat Exhaustion and Heat Stroke

Sunburn is caused by too much exposure to the ultraviolet rays of the sun. It's caused by not wearing enough protection. Sunburn can be very uncomfortable, and is serious in the case of babies and infants, whose skin is thinner than an older child's or adult's. Repeated sunburn in young children can lead to more serious problems in later life.

Signs and Symptoms

- redness or pinkness of the skin
- skin feels sore when touched
- sometimes with swelling and blistering
- sunburn can take 24 hours after exposure to reach it's worst
- fever is sometimes present
- the dead, dried skin can start to peel away after about 3 days

The worst thing you can do is to try and peel away the skin if it starts to peel. Let it come off in its own time, no matter how unsightly it is. Cool baths help a lot, especially immediately after exposure to the sun. On areas that aren't submerged in baths such as the face and neck, use cold compresses.

Baths

Run a cool bath, and add neat lavender essential oil:

Age	Essential Oil
Up to 5 years	3 drops
6 years	4 drops
7 years	5 drops
8 years	6 drops

The older your child is, add 1 extra drop per year — to a maximum of 12 drops.
If any lavender gets into the eyes, it will sting, so make sure your child is aware they should not splash about. If your child is young, stay with them to make sure they don't.

Compresses

To 1 ounce water, add 5 drops lavender essential oil. Swish the water around. Soak the compress material in this, and squeeze it out. If you place the compress over the face, make sure your child keeps their eyes closed.

The eyelids often get sunburned. For this, you could soak cotton balls in the compress water, making sure you really squeeze them out well, and place over the eye, like eye pads. Stay with your child to make sure they do not open their eyes. Repeat the compress or cotton ball methods as often as you can.

Hydrolat Compress

If you have lavender or camomile hydrolats (or "waters"), use them in the compress method. Soak the compress material in the hydolat — either lavender or camomile, or a combination of both. Squeeze out, and place gently over the burnt areas of skin.

Prepare a lot of compresses and keep them in the refrigerator. Use them throughout the day, until the child's skin has cooled down.

This method is particularly helpful in cases of sunburn on the face or eyelids — making sure the eyes are closed.

Aloe Vera

The aloe vera plant is used all over the world to soothe the skin after too much exposure to the sun. The plant grows easily and doesn't take much looking after, and you can cut a leaf anytime, to extract the gooey healing juice inside the thick hard leaves.

Mix together:

1 teaspoon aloe vera
5 drops lavender

Smear the mixture over sunburnt skin.

> ## *Calamine Lotion*
>
> *Calamine lotion is readily available, and essential oil can be added to it.*
>
> *Mix together:*
>
> *8 ounces calamine lotion*
> *10 drops camomile german*
> *30 drops lavender*
>
> *Shake the bottle well and apply to affected areas.*

Essential Oils That Help

Lavender   Camomile german
Eucalyptus radiata

Other Care

See Prevention, below.

When to Get Help

Get medical help if the skin is very sore, or if it's blistering. Also get medical help if your child has a headache or other pain, a temperature, dry mouth, or if they are shivering.

Prevention

It's important to use common sense when going in the sun with children.

- Don't take young children and infants in the sun without high factor sun screen, hats, other protective clothing, and a sunshade.
- Sun screen should not be used on babies less than 6 months old, so make sure your baby is kept out of the sunlight, and wears protective clothing.
- Put sun screen on all children in any strong sunlight. Keep all children out of strong sun between the hours of 11 A.M. to 2 P.M.
- Take adequate clothing when going in the sun, including a hat, and T-shirt to wear at the beach or swimming pool.

- Make sure your child drinks often if they are in the sun.
- After being in the sun, and whether there is redness on the skin or not, put a cooling lotion, gel, or plain water on your child's body, to cool it down.
- Teach your child the rules about going in the sun, no matter what color skin your child has, Caucasian, Asian, African-American, or mixed race. All skins can burn.

SWIMMER'S EAR (EXTERNAL OTITIS)

Swimmer's ear (or external otitis) is an inflammation in the visible part of the ear canal, caused by a bacterial or fungal infection, caught while swimming. It's less common in swimming pools that are maintained with chlorine and other chemical products used in the water. But it's common in lakes, especially during the summer, and can also be found in the ocean. External otitis can also be caught through poor hygiene — if a child touches bacteria with their hands and inserts fingers or other objects into their ears. Once a child has the infection, it seems they are more likely to be susceptible to further outbreaks.

Signs and Symptoms

- redness in ear
- itching
- pain
- fluid coming out of the ear

Ear Ointment

Mix the following together thoroughly:

$1/_2$ ounce vegetable-based ointment
10 drops camomile german
4 drops thyme linalol
4 drops palmarosa

Apply a small amount to the outer ear canal.

To make an ear plug, put a little ointment on a large piece of cotton ball — much larger than the ear hole. Tuck it just inside the ear, and leave there for at least an hour. Be careful not to push the cotton ball into the ear canal.

Essential Oils That Help

Thyme linalol   Camomile german
Palmarosa

When to Get Help

Get medical help if there is pain or discharge from the ear, if the ear seems swollen, or if your child scratches their ear a lot.

Prevention

- Don't swim in lake water if it looks murky, or when the weather is very hot and humid, or if you've heard that other people have caught infections or rashes from swimming in a particular lake.
- Before your child goes swimming, gently wipe a tiny amount of olive oil or vegetable-based (Vaseline type) ointment around the outer part of the ear and ear canal.
- Have your child wear ear plugs, or pull a swimming hat down over their ears.
- Dry the ears thoroughly after each swim, wherever that happens to be, and if there are showers, use them.

SWOLLEN LYMPH GLANDS/NODES
See also: Mononucleosis and Sore Throat

When a gland in the neck or groin swells, it means it's fighting an infection and really doing its job. The first sign of infection is often the lymph nodes swelling up, and other symptoms then follow. The lymph nodes act as a filter system, preventing bacteria, viruses, and other microorganisms from entering the blood stream. Sometimes the lymph nodes themselves become infected, preceding an infection.

Signs and Symptoms

- glands in the neck or groin area swell, or feel very sore and painful when touched
- glands in neck: throat seems red and swollen

Lymph Gland Oil

A swollen lymph node can be large and hard, or small and pea-like. Certain essential oils applied to this area will have a good chance of dealing with the infection. They are:

thyme linalol
tea tree

For children 6 years of age and over, apply 1 drop neat essential oil (either of the above), directly on the swollen lymph node: in the neck or in the groin area — being careful to avoid the genitals. If two glands are swollen, put 1 drop on each. Do this twice a day, for no longer than 3 days.

For children 5 years and under, dilute the drop of essential oil with 1 drop vegetable oil, then apply as above.

Compresses

Use the compress method in the usual way, using luke-warm water and the following essential oils:

6 drops thyme linalol
5 drops tea tree

Soak in the water, squeeze out well, and apply over the swollen area.

Essential Oils That Help

Different essential oils help, depending on the particular infection. Without knowing which particular bacteria or organism has infected your child, advice cannot be given. However, in the following list, thyme linalol is the strongest antibacterial and should be used sparingly.

Thyme linalol	Tea tree
Lavender	Camomile german
Manuka	Camomile roman

Other Care

The plant echinacea is very useful at fighting infection, and comes in different preparations. Always follow the directions on the packet. The drops are far easier to take than the tablet, especially for children, and are more easily absorbed. Increase your child's intake of vitamin C.

When to Get Help

Get help if there is a temperature or fever, sore throat, stiff neck, or rash. Get emergency medical help if there is swelling in one of the glands in the body, with no pain, which doesn't go away after 2 weeks, and there is weight loss, night sweats, tiredness, bruising, or a small, reddish-purple rash. This group of symptoms could indicate lymphoma.

TATTOOING

Human beings have been tattooing themselves since earliest historic times, despite the fact it's sometimes difficult to understand why they should want to do it. Today, tattoos are a major fashion statement, with girls as well as boys, and preteens as well as teenagers and young adults. Basically, tattooing is the insertion of permanent color under the surface of the skin using needles. Problems with infection do occasionally occur when the job is done professionally, but trouble can really start when juveniles decide it's something they can do to each other.

Tattooing is not without its risks. Equipment that has not been sterilized can transmit not only viral, bacterial, and fungal infection, but tetanus, hepatitis, and HIV. Problems can also arise because of an allergic reaction to the chemicals in the dye or ink used.

Few parents are pleased when their child comes home with a tattoo, but rather than getting highly emotional over it, take precautionary measures to ensure your child's safety. It's important to find out under what circumstances the tattooing was done. Ask whether the needles were sterilized, and in which way. If you feel there may be a major risk, consult your doctor. In other cases, apply the measures below.

If infection has already occurred, visit your doctor immediately due to the risks involved. In adulthood, dermabrasion and laser treatment can be used to remove tattoos, but they usually leave some degree of scarring.

To Help Prevent Infection

First wash the area with a strong disinfectant solution. Then mix together:

20 drops thyme linalol
20 drops lavender
20 drops tea tree

From this blend of neat essential oils, apply 1 drop over each square inch of the affected area, to a maximum of 5 drops. Leave to dry. Repeat as often as possible over the coming week.

Essential Oils That Help

Thyme linalol

Lavender

Tea tree

Camomile german

Manuka

Niaouli

Elemi

Parent's Tip

If your child has been pressured at school into having a tattoo and doesn't really want it, try wiping the area with neat lemon, orange, or grapefruit essential oil. These oils can cause skin irritation because they are photosensitive; the skin shouldn't be exposed to sunlight while the oils are on it. But if used directly after home tattooing, these citrus oils often help fade the markings. If not available, try lemon juice.

TEETHING

Babies usually start teething from the age of 6 months. By the time they're 2 years of age, twenty "milk" teeth will have emerged from the gums. Some teeth will have difficulty coming through, and cause soreness and pain. To find out if your child is teething, look to see if there are inflamed areas on the gum and, with a very clean finger, feel around the gums for hard bumps. If you find either of these things, the likelihood is that baby is teething.

Signs and Symptoms

- dribbling, rashes around the mouth
- biting on anything, baby trying to put fist in the mouth
- can be: fever, runny stools
- difficulty sleeping, crying, irritability

Above all, at this time, babies need reassuring with cuddles and comfort. Adopt the classic pose of a parent with a teething child — walking up and down, patting their back, saying "there, there."

Cold Compresses

Apply cool compresses over the jaw area, made using:

lavender hydrolat/ "water"
camomile hydrolat/ "water"

See pages 11–12 for how hydrolats or essential oil "waters" are made. Dip a folded piece of muslin into the hydolat or "water," squeeze it out well, and lay along baby's jawline.

To Help Sleep Oil

First mix the following together:

1 dessertspoon vegetable oil
1 drop petitgrain
1 drop lavender

Rub a small amount of the diluted oil over the back, the back of the neck, and the soles of the feet.

Essential Oils That Help

Camomile german   Cardamom
Camomile roman   Eucalyptus radiata

Essential Oils That Help for Calming and Sleep

Lavender
Petitgrain

Other Care

Homeopathic camomile teething granules may help. Give your child soothing, soft, cool, foods such as yogurt, ice cream, and Jell-O. Teething rings help the soreness — keep them in the refrigerator, not the freezer. If you give your baby peeled apple or carrot to gnaw on, make sure you stay with them.

When to Get Help

Get help if your baby has any symptoms you are worried about.

THRUSH (CANDIDA ALBICANS) — YEAST INFECTION

See also: Diaper Rash

Yeasts are a type of fungus. One type of fungus is the yeast, Candida Albicans, that can flourish almost anywhere within the gastrointestinal tract — of babies, children, and adults alike. It can infect the mouth, throat, stomach, intestines, anus and, in girls, the vagina and vulva area. This yeast (or fungal) infection is often called "thrush" or "candidiasis."

Babies can catch thrush during labor from their mother's birth canal, or it can be caught anytime afterward from infected breast nipples, or feeding bottles. Children who have generally low resistance are at risk, as are those who have been on long courses of antibiotics — which not only kill off targeted unfriendly bacteria, but the normal friendly bacteria that live in a healthy intestinal tract. When there are no longer enough friendly bacteria to fight off the yeast infection, it's left free to become rampant.

Signs and Symptoms

- whitish, cream-colored frothy creamy patches on: the roof of the mouth, gums, inner cheeks, tongue, and sometimes on the lips
- the child may refuse to eat
- creamy patches around the anus, and, in girls, possibly around the vaginal and vulva area
- a rash similar to a diaper rash, a pimple filled red patch
- the rash spots can cause sores if the outer, white coating is rubbed off

Anal Washing

Use either of the methods below, to help keep infection and irritation in the area under control.

Yogurt Method	Tea Wash Method
Stir together well:	Prepare a tea using:
1 ounce carton plain, unflavored, bioactive yogurt 5 drops tea tree 3 drops camomile german 5 drops palmarosa	$^1/_2$ pint water 5 drops tea tree 5 drops palmarosa 5 drops camomile german
Use a tiny amount to spread around the anal area — after each diaper change, or after using the toilet.	Use the tea to wash or wipe the anal area after each diaper change, or after using the toilet. Bioactive natural yogurt can also be added to this tea.

Baths

If the genital area has become infected, use the other methods in this section and, when your child has a bath, add to the water:

1 teaspoon bicarbonate of soda

Body Oil

The following mix can be diluted in vegetable oil to make a body oil. Use it over the whole body, avoiding the face and genital area. See pages 15–31 for instructions on how many drops of the mix to use, depending on the age of your child.

First mix together:

10 drops tea tree
6 drops camomile german
6 drops palmarosa

Mouthwash

Only use this method if your child's mouth is affected. Only use it with children who are old enough to use a mouthwash and spit it out afterward.

Prepare a tea using:

$^1/_2$ pint water
5 drops tea tree
5 drops palmarosa
5 drops camomile german

Pour the tea through an unbleached paper coffee filter and bottle. To prepare the mouthwash, mix together:

1 dessertspoon filtered tea
$^1/_4$ pint water
1 dessertspoon unflavored bioactive yogurt

Have your child use this as a mouthwash, making sure they spit it out afterward.

Essential Oils That Help

Tea tree   Manuka
Camomile german   Palmarosa
Thyme linalol   Geranium
Patchouli

Other Care

To stop the infection spreading from the mouth to the genital area, and visa versa, make sure your child washes their hands before and after using the bathroom. If your child is a baby, leave their diapers off as much as possible.

Give your infant cool foods to help soothe the mouth. The best choice would be unflavored, unsweetened, bioactive yogurt — the type that has active friendly bacteria in it. Avoid all products with sugar in them as the fungus thrives on a diet of sugar. Encourage older children to avoid eating dairy products, wheat products, and foods that contain yeast. Consider giving your child acidophilus supplements. See also Prevention, below.

When to Get Help

Get help as soon as you suspect your child has thrush.

Prevention

See Other Care, above. Good hygiene is essential to help prevent your baby being infected with thrush.

- Before feeding your baby from the breast, wash the nipple area. If going out and about, take a sterile wipe with you, and use to wipe the nipple before placing it in the baby's mouth.
- If you bottle feed your baby, wash your hands before preparing feeds. Make sure you first boil, then sterilize, all bottle nipples.
- Public bathrooms sometimes provide diaper changing facilities, however, this is not the place to feed your baby as bacteria from fecal matter can be airborne.

TONSILLITIS

See also: Sore Throat

Tonsillitis is inflammation of the tonsils, usually caused by the bacteria streptococcus, but sometimes by a virus. The adenoids may also become infected. The tonsils are two patches on either side, right at the back of the throat, and can be seen when the child opens their mouth very wide. As part of the lymphatic system, the job of the tonsils is to help fight infection by trapping germs and preventing them from entering the respiratory system and other parts of the body. Tonsils often become enlarged when a child is fighting an infection. Tonsillitis is more common in children of school age.

Signs and Symptoms

- sore throat, difficulty in swallowing
- tonsils seem red — inflammation, may have white spots of pus on them
- temperature may go over 100°F
- bad breath, or snoring during sleep
- headache, earache, neckache, or tummy ache
- chills, or cough

To see if your child's tonsils are infected, get them to open their mouth wide, and hold the tongue down with a tongue depressor, or the back of the handle of a spoon. Tell your child to say "aaah." As they do this, you'll be able to see more of the throat. Check your child's temperature, and feel either side of their neck to see if the glands are swollen.

Glands Oil

Put a couple of drops pure thyme linalol essential oil on your fingertips and apply over the glands on either side of the neck. Then gently wipe a little vegetable oil over the top. Repeat before sleep every night.

Tonsillitis Compress and Oil Mix

This mix was published in one of my earlier books and I know from the many letters I've received that it's been very effective. This is a two-part method.

First mix the essential oils together:

10 drops lavender
15 drops tea tree
5 drops ginger
2 drops lemon

Warm Compress

Use 4 drops of the tonsillitis mix in the compress method. Put warm water in a bowl, add the essential oils, put a cloth in the water, squeeze it out, and place it over the throat area. Do this twice a day.

Abdomen and Back Oil

Mix together:

1 dessertspoon vegetable oil
5 drops tonsillitis mix

Using a small amount each time, apply over the upper abdomen and upper back.

Gargle

This method can only be used by children who are old enough to gargle and spit out afterward. Use only 1 teaspoon in a glass of warm water for a gargle.

First mix together:

1 ounce pure spring water
3 tablespoons cider vinegar
3 drops ginger
5 drops lemon

Stir everything together, then pour through an unbleached paper coffee filter. Then mix in:

1 tablespoon honey

Stir the honey in well, until the liquid is all one consistency, then bottle.
Put 1 teaspoon of the final mix in a small glass of warm water, and use as a gargle. Do this twice a day.

Rose Syrup

This syrup goes down like a treat when the tonsils are sore. This is what you will need:

enough fragrant, organically grown, rose petals to fill a pint jar
1 pound organic brown granulated sugar
1 pint spring water
the juice of 1 lemon
3 drops rose otto essential oil

Wash the rose petals thoroughly in water. Put the spring water into a small cooking pot, with the rose petals. Cover the pot with a lid and bring to a boil. Turn the heat down, so the pot can simmer very gently for 10 minutes. Then turn the heat off completely, but leave the pot right where it is, for another two hours. Strain the mixture, then top off the water level until it's back to one pint again. Add the lemon juice, the essential oil drops, and the sugar. Stir slowly until it thickens, then pour into jars.

Honey is very soothing for all types of sore throat. The same method can be used substituting 1 pound of honey for 1 pound of sugar. Use very thick set honey.

Essential Oils That Help

Lavender   Tea tree
Thyme linalol   Lemon
Ginger   Camomile roman
Camomile german

Other Care

Give your child soothing drinks. Use warm compresses over the throat area. Keep the air circulating in your child's room.

When to Get Help

If your child is a small baby, contact your pediatrician as soon as you suspect tonsillitis. With all other children, get medical help if your child can't swallow properly, if they have a high fever, complain of earache, or if the condition generally seems to be getting worse.

TOOTHACHE

Pain in the area of the teeth can be caused by tooth decay, gum infection, biting on a hard object, or an injury to a tooth.

Signs and Symptoms

- pain in the tooth or gum
- earache
- a tooth problem can be felt as face ache; the face may become swollen — often a sign of abscess
- drinking or eating something cold, hot, or sweet, causes pain — a sign of tooth decay
- red and swollen gums — a sign of an abscess or gum boil

Jaw Oil

Mix together the following:

1 teaspoon vegetable oil
1 drop clove
1 drop helichrysum
3 drops camomile german

Rub a little of the diluted oil along the external jaw line.

Compresses

Use warm water or, if the child prefers it, ice cold water. Put 1 ounce water in a small bowl and add:

2 drops camomile roman

Soak the compress material in the water, squeeze out, and apply to the painful side of the jaw.

> ## Mouth Rinses and Rubs
>
> *Only use this method with children over 5 years of age. The child must be able to rinse the mouth, then spit the liquid out. Use tincture of myrrh, available from drug stores, and follow directions on the packaging.*
>
> ☜
>
> *For infected gums, make your own myrrh tincture by adding 2 drops myrrh essential oil to 1 teaspoon consumable alcohol, such as brandy or vodka, and 1 dessertspoon water. Put it all into a dropper bottle. When ready for use, put just one drop of the mix into 1 teaspoon warm water. Dip a cotton ball into this mixture, and use it to rub gently around the gum. Use a clean cotton ball each time. If gum boils are present, add 1 drop thyme linalol to the above mix.*

Essential Oils That Help

Camomile roman	Camomile german
Clove	Helichrysum
Lemon	Myrrh

Other Care

Ice packs or cold compresses may help reduce the swelling. Pain can sometimes be relieved by warmth applied to the area, such as in warm compresses, or by a warm towel or hot water bottle being held against the affected side of the face. Check the lymph glands to see if they are swollen. See Swollen Lymph Glands/Nodes.

When to Get Help

Consult your dentist to prevent tooth decay and other problems. See your doctor if there has been any facial injury.

Prevention

- Regular visits to the dentist will help identify any potential problems.
- Teach your child to brush their teeth correctly, and to floss after eating and before bedtime. Visit an oral hygienist, who can teach your child proper dental hygiene habits.
- Cut down on candy intake, sweet foods, and sodas.

- Give your child water to drink after eating candy and other sweets, to flush through the sugar.
- Do not give young children bottles of juice at bedtime — even pure fruit juice. After they've brushed their teeth, only give them water.
- Give drinks to small children in a plastic beaker-type cup, with a lid, and mouthpiece that is long enough to bypass the teeth.

TUBERCULOSIS — "TB"

Although rare, TB is on the increase. It's caused by the bacteria *Mycobacterium tuberculosis*. TB used to be spread through the milk of infected cows, but today it's usually caught by breathing in the moisture put into the atmosphere by infected people coughing or sneezing. TB mostly affects the lungs, but can involve all the organs of the body when spread through the blood stream. There are various forms of TB that can be identified by a simple skin test.

Signs and Symptoms

- no symptoms except flu-like symptoms — often mistaken for flu, children with recurrent bouts of flu should be checked for TB
- persistent dry cough
- nighttime sweating
- possibly: blood in the sputum
- chest pain
- headache, lack of appetite, lack of energy, weight loss, fever

Tuberculosis (TB) Mix
This mix can be used in the two methods below. Follow the instructions in each box. First mix the following essential oils together: 10 drops thyme linalol 10 drops ravensara 10 drops niaouli

Body Oil	Warm Baths
From the TB mix, take double the number of drops recommended for your child's age on pages 15–31, and add to: 1/2 ounce vegetable oil Use the oil to rub over the whole of your child's body, twice a day. This amount will be enough for several applications, depending on the size of your child.	From the TB mix, take the number of drops recommended for your child's age on pages 15–31, and add to: 1 teaspoon vegetable oil Put in the bath water, and swish around well before your child gets in.

Essential Oils That Help

In Diffuser or Other Room Methods only

Ravensara

Niaouli

Thyme linalol

Eucalyptus radiata

Oregano

Cinnamon

Clove

Other Care

Your child will need plenty of rest, and a good diet of home cooking, with a multivitamin supplement. Your child may have to be absent from school for several months, so keep them occupied with home study activities, by liasing with their teachers. Your child will not be infectious once drug treatment from your doctor has been started. Once drug treatment has started, they can play with other children.

When to Get Help

Inform your doctor as soon as possible if any of the above symptoms occur. Get medical advice if your child has been in the company of anyone with TB.

Prevention

- Inoculations are available.
- A skin test can determine whether your child has TB.

UMBILICAL CORD INFECTION

At birth, the umbilical cord is clamped and cut, and over the next week to ten days the remaining stump shrivels up, then falls off. It can become infected if cleaning is not carried out correctly, or if urine or fecal matter have seeped into the area.

Signs and Symptoms

- redness and swelling together
- fluid weeping from the stump
- crusting over, pus
- after the cord drops off: a discharge from the area is a sign of infection

---

Cleaning Methods

Newborn babies have very thin skin, as it has yet to mature. Only use very small amounts of anything on the skin.

Cleansing Wash	Cotton Ball Method
First put 1 drop lavender into a teaspoon of salt, and add to the water you are going to use for washing. Then pour through an unbleached paper coffee filter. Now use to gently bathe the area.	*First wash your hands. Put 1 drop lavender onto a cotton ball. Dip the cotton ball in a cup of water, squeeze the excess water out between your fingertips. Use the cotton ball to carefully clean around the area. Do this twice a day.*

Neat Oil

Use this method if your baby's umbilical cord clearly has signs of infection. First wash your hands. Smear a tiny amount neat lavender oil (less than 1 drop) on one of your fingertips, and wipe that fingertip in a circle around the base of the stump, taking care not to touch any infected or cut area.

Essential Oils That Help

Tea tree   Lavender
Camomile german

Other Care

Wipe the cord after each diaper change. This can be carried out using surgical spirit. Use a little salt water in the baby's bath, and also bathe the area with salt water. Always let the stump fall off naturally, so a nice belly button is formed.

When to Get Help

Get help if the stump seems red or swollen, or there is a discharge.

Prevention

- Always check the cord stump at each diaper change.
- As often as possible, leave the umbilical area exposed to the air to help it dry up.

URINARY TRACT INFECTION

Urinary tract infection is usually caused by a bacteria in the urinary system, but can also be caused by viral or fungal infection. It can affect the kidneys, ureters, bladder, and urethra. Cystitis is the most common type of urinary tract infection, but there are others, such as urethritis and pyelonephritis.

Signs and Symptoms
- can occur in girls and boys, often occurs in uncircumcized male children
- burning sensation when passing urine
- strongly colored, strong-smelling urine
- feeling the frequent need of urination, often with just a dribble
- back pain may be located just above the waist-line
- may be: tummy pain, feeling nauseous, vomiting
- in children who were previously dry at night — bed-wetting (as the body tries to rid itself of the infection)

Warm Baths

Dilute 3 drops tea tree in 1 teaspoon vegetable oil, and add to the warm bath water. Also add 1 teaspoon salt to the water. Swish around well before the child gets in.

Urinary Tract Mix

The following mix can be used in the three methods below. Follow the directions in each box. First mix the following together:

5 drops niaouli
5 drops tea tree
5 drops bergamot
5 drops mandarin
6 drops camomile german

Warm Compresses	Body Oil for the Back	Boy's Wash
Apply warm compresses over your child's back, just above the waist line. Put $^1/_2$ pint warm water in a bowl and add: 5 drops of the urinary tract infection mix Soak the compress material in the water, squeeze out, and apply.	See page 16 for the number of drops of essential oil to use for your child's age, in the body rub method. Use the appropriate number of drops of the urinary tract infection mix, diluted in the appropriate amount of vegetable oil. Gently rub over the lower back.	Put the following in a clean bowl: $^1/_2$ pint luke-warm water 1 teaspoon salt 5 drops of the urinary tract infection mix Swish the water around well, and use to bathe the penis. Gently pull back the foreskin and wash the area underneath.

Essential Oils That Help

Tea tree	Bergamot
Niaouli	Lavender
Camomile german	

Other Care

Give your child plenty of pure, unadulterated cranberry juice, as this helps to clear up urinary infection. Freeze-dried powdered cranberry can be used by older children. If no cranberry juice is available, buy frozen cranberries and cook them in water. Then put the cranberries and cooking water into a blender, adding enough additional water to make a juice. Sieve the juice before giving it to your child. Do not add sugar at any point in the process.

Increase your child's water intake; they should not be given any gaseous or sugar-laden drinks. Don't let them use bubble bath or other bath preparations — only use diluted essential oils in the bath. Put your child in pure cotton underwear. Warm compresses, hot water bottles, or warmed towels placed over the area of the kidneys often helps — apply on the back, just above the waist.

When to Get Help

Get medical help if your child complains of pain when passing urine, if the urine smells unusually unpleasant; or if it is cloudy, or very strongly colored. Also, get help if your child is itchy in the area, or feels the need to pass urine frequently, but cannot do so.

Prevention

- Teach girls that after urinating, they should wipe from the front of the genital area toward the back.

VOMITING

See also: Dehydration

When food or fluid is regurgitated from the stomach, it's called vomiting. Vomiting is one of the ways the body rids itself of infection or toxins that have entered the body, usually in the form of a bacteria or other microorganisms. If the vomiting is serious, it can lead to dehydration.

Babies and infants often regurgitate their food, and this is nothing to worry about, unless it becomes continuous, where your child holds nothing down. But when a child of any age has what's known as projectile vomiting, there is something to worry about. This is when food or liquid is thrown up with such force it lands several feet away. Projectile vomiting is caused by a muscular abnormality, and must be seen by a physician as soon as possible. Insist that your child is given a thorough examination.

Signs and Symptoms

- uncontrollable regurgitating of food or liquid through the mouth

Vomiting Mix	
Use the following essential oils in equal amounts in the two methods below: lavender camomile roman	

Compress	Tissue or Pillow
Use only on children over 2 years of age. Put a pint of cool or luke-warm water in a bowl, and add 2 drops each lavender and camomile roman essential oil. Swish around well. Put a cloth in the water, and squeeze it out well. Ask your child to close their eyes, then place the compress over their forehead.	Mix together a couple of drops lavender and camomile roman essential oil, using equal amounts. Use one of these methods: Put 1 drop of the mix on a tissue and give it to your child to sniff. Put 1 drop on your child's pillow — on the underside, away from the eyes. Lay your child down to rest. The essential oils will calm your child if they're fretful, and help them to sleep.

Essential Oils That Help

Ginger	Peppermint
Spearmint	Lavender

Other Care

Do not attempt to stop the vomiting. When your child is vomiting, hold their forehead steady, and pull their hair out of the way. After each bout of vomiting, wash your child's face gently with cool or luke-warm water. You could also place a cool wet flannel or a compress over your child's forehead, or on the back of their neck, to cool them down and generally make them feel better.

Give your child nothing to eat or drink until at least one hour after the vomiting has stopped. Then give them a small glass of plain, boiled water, which has been cooled, and ask them to take small sips continuously.

When to Get Help

Get help immediately if there are: stomach cramps, fever, headache, coughing, or if the vomiting continues for longer than 5 hours.

Prevention

- Don't try to prevent vomiting. It's best to let the body rid itself of whatever it needs to.

WARTS

Warts are caused by the virus *human papillomavirus,* and are benign skin growths. They are transmitted by direct contact, and can be contracted in public places if touching a surface after an infected person has touched it. There are several types including hand warts, the so-called "plantar" warts that attach themselves to the feet, and "flat" warts that grow on the face.

Sexually active teenagers are at risk of genital warts that can appear on the penis or vulva area. Girls with genital warts are at risk of cervical cancer, and genital warts in boys as well as in girls, must be treated immediately by a doctor.

Signs and Symptoms

- **Hand Warts**

  These grow on the child's hand or fingers — usually on the back of the hand, the fingers, and around the fingernail. They start out as small bumps, often pinkish in color. They're elevated above the surface of the flesh, and have a scaly surface. Sometimes there's a horn-type of protrusion. These often disappear all by themselves in time.

- **Plantar Warts**

  Plantar warts grow on the feet, and the infection is often picked up walking around swimming pools, gyms, and showers. The wart has a central core which starts out soft but gradually grows into a hard, horny surface area, level with the flesh. They have a distinct core, which is often marked by a black spot. This spot is made up of blood vessels.

- **Flat Warts**

  Flat warts can grow on a child's face, and are called 'flat' because they are much smoother than other types of wart, and close to the surface of the skin. Although generally smaller than other types of wart, flat warts can grow in groups of as many as twenty. Facial warts should only be treated by a doctor.

The following recommendations are only for warts on the hand and fingers, or plantar warts on the feet or toes.

<table>
<tr><td colspan="2" align="center">

Hand, Finger, Foot, and Toe Wart Mix

</td></tr>
<tr><td colspan="2">

Use this mix in either of the two methods below. First mix the following essential oils together:

10 drops lemon
5 drops bergamot
2 drops cypress
5 drops manuka
4 drops thyme red
1 drop clove

</td></tr>
<tr><td>

Hand and Finger Warts

</td><td>

Plantar Warts — Feet and Toes

</td></tr>
<tr><td>

This method can only be used if your child can be guaranteed not to put their hand anywhere near their mouth or face. Dip a clean Q-tip into the wart mix and dab a small amount of the mix directly on the wart. Use only once a day, for no more than 10 days.

</td><td>

Dip a clean Q-tip into the wart mix and dab a small amount of the mix directly on the wart. Do this twice a day, for no more than 10 days.

</td></tr>
</table>

Essential Oils That Help

Lemon   Bergamot
Cypress   Manuka
Thyme linalol   *Dermatect (See Suppliers)

When to Get Help

Get help if the wart is bleeding, or if your child is scratching the wart and there's a risk of infection. Take advice if the wart doesn't disappear after 8 weeks. Also, get help if the wart is swollen or becomes red or if, for any reason, either you or the child are worried. A doctor can freeze or laser the warts off.

WHOOPING COUGH

Whooping cough is a highly contagious disease caused by the bacteria *bordatelle pertussis*. It affects the respiratory system, with the airways becoming blocked with mucus. The most characteristic symptom is a high-pitched "whoop" sound made as the air tries to pass through a swollen larynx during a coughing bout. Whooping cough can last up to eight weeks, during which time the child is especially vulnerable to pneumonia or bronchitis (see pages 216 and 84), as well as other serious conditions.

Signs and Symptoms

- starts with cold-like symptoms that last 10 to 14 days
- then the cough starts
- cough — with or without the "whoop" sound
- difficulty in breathing while coughing
- vomiting, particularly after a coughing bout
- disturbed sleep, tiredness, irritability, crying

Baths	*Chest Rub*
Dilute the following essential oils in 1 teaspoon vegetable oil:	Use a small amount of the following mix, over the chest and back, before sleep every night:
3 drops thyme linalol 1 drop lavender 1 drop niaouli	1 ounce almond oil 15 drops thyme linalol 15 drops ravensara 20 drops lavender
Add the diluted oil to the bath water, and swish around well before your child gets in.	

Whooping Cough Mix

The following mix can be used in the two methods below. Follow the instructions in the boxes.

First mix the following:

10 drops thyme linalol
10 drops ravensara
10 drops eucalyptus radiata

Steaming Bowls	Pillow
Put 10 drops of the whooping cough mix in a small bowl of steaming hot water. Place the bowl in your child's room, somewhere out of reach of children and pets. Keep the door closed.	At night, put 2 drops of the whooping cough mix on your child's pillow — on the underside, away from their eyes. It may stain, so use an old pillowcase. To help with the coughing, prop your child upright on lots of extra pillows.

Essential Oils That Help

Thyme linalol	Eucalyptus radiata
Ravensara	Cypress
Lavender	* Dermatect (See Suppliers)

Professional aromatherapists may want to add one of the following three to this list: Hyssopus decumbrens — add 2 to 3 drops to the whooping cough mix above, or, alternatively, add 4 drops Thymus vulgaris, or 4 drops origanum vulgare.

Other Care

Fresh air is needed, so open a window. Use a humidifier in your child's room. Keep them away from atmospheric pollution, including cigarette smoke. Give your child lots to drink to rehydrate their body (see Dehydration). Only give your child small meals, in case food is brought up during a bout of coughing. Fish, chicken, and green vegetables are what they need now — liquified into a soup if that's the only way they'll eat it. Also give your child vitamin C, and cod liver oil.

Mucus and phlegm will be coughed up. Keep a bowl nearby so your child can spit into it. Sterilize the bowl continually with boiling water and bleach.

Don't send your child back to school or kindergarten until you have the approval of their doctor.

When to Get Help

Whooping cough can be very serious in young children. Speak to your doctor immediately if you suspect whooping cough, especially if you know someone in the neighborhood, or school, has it.

Prevention

- Inoculation is available; ask your doctor about vaccinations.

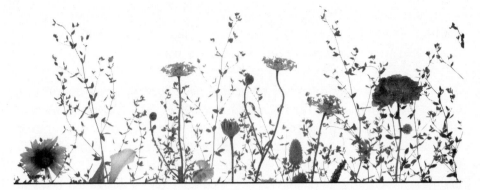

CHAPTER FIVE **The Seriously Ill Child**

There are children who have been loved and cared for, and even prayed for most intently, who will become seriously ill and, tragically, some may not recover. Their parents will go through heart-breaking agony, often accompanied by feelings of guilt ("I didn't do enough"), fear ("how much more pain will my child have to suffer"), depression and sadness ("I cannot go on without my child"). At the same time, they're expected to be stoic and positive, for the sake of their child. Parents have told me they loathed the feeling of exclusion, as they stood in corridors while strangers, the professionals, carried on their business around their child's bed.

We are very grateful to the doctors and nurses who care for our sick children, and there is no substitute for what they do. Many doctors today are aiming to integrate conventional medical treatment with the best of the complementary therapies. It's called "integrative medicine." Aromatherapy is very much at the forefront of this trend, and not only because people find it so very pleasant, with its delicious aromas. Hospitals and hospices in many countries have trained aromatherapy staff on the premises. To suggest using a few essential oils on your child is not going to surprise many medical staff; they've probably seen it done before.

Using essential oils on a sick child is one way to contribute toward their care. It does generally make children feel more comfortable. The lovely aromas lift the spirits, and bring the richness of nature into the environment. As they allay fears and anxiety, they may also introduce a new positivity. It's fairly easy to use aromatherapy within a medical care environment. Essential oil sprays can be used in the atmosphere, and around bed linen. If your child is at home, rather than a medical facility, a diffuser could be used.

When it comes to massage, you need medical clearance from your child's doctor. They will want to consider whether the delivery of drugs they've prescribed will be affected by the increased blood flow. Each patient is different. It may be possible to massage your child's hands, or feet, arms, legs, or even their back. It may be more suitable to stroke their forehead, or their head. A simple hand massage would be a good place to start, because it leads on so naturally from that thing all parents with sick children do — sit by their bed and hold their hand. Just put a little oil on your child's hand and stroke it in gently, or massage very lightly.

Essential Oils for the Seriously Ill Child

The dilution rates are $^1/_3$ *lower for sick children than for healthy children, unless carried out by a professional.*

rose otto	neroli	lemon
camomile roman	lavender	mandarin
tangerine	orange	geranium
		petitgrain

Massage

Massage can increase blood flow, and this can have an impact on the way carefully measured doses of drugs are delivered through the body — in chemotherapy, for example. For this reason, most institutions would prefer you to ask before attempting to massage your child.

By "massage" I'm talking about very gentle upward movements, more like stroking, over and over again, on different parts of the body. If you are unsure, the hands and feet are a good place to start.

Room Sprays

Essential oils can be used in room sprays to freshen up the stale air that is often present in hospitals. Don't let the water droplets fall on any electrical equipment. Choose from the suitable oils above. A little lavender can help a child to sleep. See page 21 in Methods for the quantities to use with different age groups and method instructions.

Drug Dependent Babies

I'll never forget hearing from a pediatric nurse that the worst thing about caring for drug-dependent babies is the constant crying and screaming of innocent little souls going through withdrawal. Each baby is born with their particular set of symptoms and problems, possibly including infection with HIV. The nurses often feel helpless, and I know that for some it's just too much to cope with emotionally — especially as, for crack-dependent babies, the out-look is not always good. Medication is of course given to these unfortunate children, and the best care, including being picked up, cuddled, and soothed.

Aromatherapy can help in terms of emotional soothing, and taking some of the edge off the harsh physical effects of withdrawal. A baby who has been subjected to narcotic drugs while in the womb, and is now on medication, must be treated with a different set of rules to babies who haven't had to endure this unnatural assault on their system.

Drug Dependent Babies

The following essential oils are suitable for use on drug dependent babies:

lavender
neroli
camomile roman
rose otto

Each baby will have a smell preference which, with patience, you may discover.

For newborns, in whom the symptoms of withdrawal are at their worse, use 3 drops essential oil, diluted in ¹/₂ ounce almond oil. Gradually *reduce* the amount of essential oil over the following weeks, until the minimum amount of essential oil recommended for that age group is being used. Apply the diluted oil in a very gentle massage of the back, arms, and legs. As these babies are always underweight, only a tiny amount will actually be used. Remember to be extremely gentle when applying the oil.

The same essential oil as used in the soothing massage can also be placed near the baby — just one drop placed on a tissue. The aroma will remind the baby of the love and care given to them with the gentle soothing massage, and bring some reassurance and calm. Only use the same oil or blend of oils you are using in the massage, if it's been established through observation that the child is benefiting from it. Signs to look for are less crying and more calm.

Healing Touch

In some forms of energy healing, the hands touch the body. In other forms they do not. Strange as it may seem, just hovering the hands, palm down, about two inches from the surface of the body, can have a very calming effect, and improve healing time. The "no hands" approach to healing can be useful when a child is on a drip, attached to other equipment, and generally in a delicate position. Simply place your hands in the air above your child, almost stroking the air around them, not touching the body itself. If your child has a tummy pain, hold your hands above the tummy. If it's in the foot, put your hands there.

What follows is a brief outline of a particular healing method taught to nurses all over the world by Dolores Kreiger Ph.D., R.N. It can be used by all parents, even those whose children are too sick to have physical contact.

First, get yourself comfortable and take a deep breath. Imagine your child at their funniest and most playful, when they were well. Keeping this image in your mind, imagine a band of energy, like the flow of a gentle stream, circling up the front of your child's body, and over their back in a never-ending, continuous movement. Then see this flow as sparkling and full of light — rather like rippling water in bright sunlight. Now join the two images together — your happy, well child, and this sparkling flow of energy, or water — whichever is the easiest for you to imagine. See the sparkling stream flowing around your child in bed. This can be difficult to do, but take your time.

The next step is to put a hand into that imaginary flow of sparkling energy and gently hold it over whichever part of the body seems to you to be the most problematic for your child at that particular time. Don't attempt to treat the illness itself, that is not your role here.

Now imagine your hand is getting full of soothing light. People will have different ideas about where the healing light comes from. Hold your hand there just for a few seconds at first, building up to a longer time later on. As soon as your mind wanders, slowly take your hand away, leaving the sparkling energy in its place.

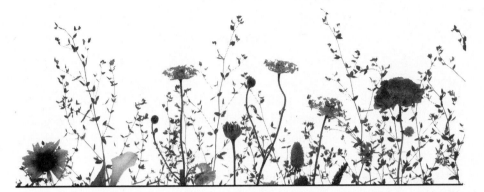

CHAPTER SIX **Mind, Mood, and Emotion**

Children can suffer with negative states of mind, just as adults can. They too can feel stress, tension, anxiety, depression, guilt, shame, and embarrassment. They too can lack self-confidence or self-esteem, and feel unworthy. Insecurity and fear may be in their mind. The pressures on children are different from the pressures on adults, but are equally tough. We have work and bills to worry about, they have homework every night, and exams every year. While we have control over our lives, and can make decisions to change what is getting us down, children do not. And control, or the lack of it, is known from research to be one of the most important factors in the build up of stress. Teenagers in particular have powerful peer pressure bending them this way and that, and the "fashion police" to watch out for.

Sometimes, tragically, the pressures on children lead them to commit suicide as a means of escape. For others, escape may be found in drugs, alcohol, belonging to a gang, or teen sex. The mental state of our children is just as important as their physical state of health, but you can't measure self-esteem on a thermometer. A rash you can see and a swollen gland you can feel, but what happens inside a child's head is hidden.

There are many subjects that come under the general title "mind, mood and emotion," and I have written about them at length in *The Fragrant Mind*. What follows is a few brief suggestions, adapted from that book.

Alertness

Children have a great deal of studying to do, and it's a strain. Keeping the mind alert through lessons and homework is hard, especially when it's a subject your child has no interest in whatsoever. When a person studies, their mind is absorbing information. The problem often with exams is in being able to actually remember the information that was studied the night before. This is where essential oils come in. When your child is studying, they can use a particular essential oil nearby, in a diffuser or on a tissue they can occasionally sniff from. The information studied then becomes associated with that particular aroma. When the exam comes along, your child can use that same aroma nearby, not in a diffuser, but on a tissue. They can discreetly sniff the aroma, which takes their mind back to study-time and may help them recall the information. There are several rules to follow in this process:

1) Try to use a fragrance the child has not used before because an aroma used previously probably has associations that have nothing to do with the subject being absorbed. Or make a unique mix especially for each subject.

2) If possible use one fragrance (or mix) per subject, and not too much.

3) Your child should only inhale the aroma when they need to remember the studied information — in a test or exam for example, and not at other times. If they use it all the time, their memory will get confused.

4) Don't rely solely on this method. The aroma-memory connection is meant to be an additional aid, not a replacement for hard work. Your child can't just look at their text books expecting everything to magically go in. Sorry, it's not that easy. They'll have to put the time in and read their material thoroughly.

Children's Alertness Oils		
peppermint	*pine*	*bergamot*
eucalyptus radiata	*lemon*	*rosemary*
grapefruit	*lime*	

Children's Alertness Mix

First, mix the following essential oils together. From this mix take the appropriate number of drops for your child's age (see pages 15–31). Use in the diffuser and tissue methods.

5 drops grapefruit
5 drops lime
2 drops black pepper
2 drops peppermint

Anxiety

You can guess your child is anxious if you find them sighing a lot, gasping for breath, or needing to take in large chunks of air. It might even be that they're running to the toilet all the time, getting headaches or back pain, biting their nails, or just can't relax. Yet tiredness is common, or restlessness, even tremors. Anxiety can make people dizzy, perspire or blush, and it can raise blood pressure. A child might feel dry in the mouth, or belch a lot, feel nauseous, get diarrhea, or vomit. The stomach muscles can tighten up in a spasm, causing terrible pain. Anxiety causes stabbing pains in the chest, and stronger, faster heartbeats. It can make a child feel so unwell their parents seriously wonder if there isn't something physical wrong.

Children's Anxiety Oils

bergamot	mandarin	neroli
rose otto	camomile roman	geranium
frankincense		

Children's Anxiety Mix

First, mix the following essential oils together. From this mix take the appropriate number of drops for your child's age (see pages 15–22). Use in baths, body oils, and all room methods.

5 drops bergamot
1 drop lavender
3 drops geranium

Stress

Children's stress can arise from exam pressure, emotional problems, peer pressure, home life difficulties, school competition pressure, high parental expectations, feelings of being unable to cope, feeling helpless, and everything being out of their control, including themselves.

Symptoms include irritability, loss of sense of humor, difficulty in making decisions or concentrating, or doing jobs in logical order, feeling defensive, angry inside and disinterested in large areas of life. Also, there may be insomnia, sweating, breathlessness, fainting, loss of appetite and bingeing, indigestion, constipation or diarrhea, headaches, cramps, muscle spasms, eczema, asthma, psoriasis, and breathing problems.

Children's Stress Oils

lavender	ormenis flower (camomile maroc)	petitgrain
camomile roman	geranium	mandarin
rose otto	neroli	ylang ylang

Children's Stress Mix

Mix the following essential oils together. From this mix take the appropriate number of drops for your child's age (see pages 15–22). Use in baths, body oils, and all room methods.

5 drops camomile roman
2 drops mandarins
3 drops ormenis flower (camomile maroc)
3 drops geranium

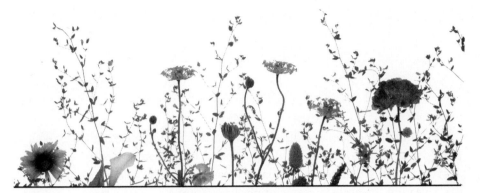

Suppliers

If you experience difficulty finding pure essential oils suitable for the purposes outlined in this book, the following aromatherapy suppliers can be recommended. The company has an international mail order following providing certified organic, wild crafted, and controlled cultivation essential oils and also supply products especially for children, babies, and mothers-to-be.

Details of the author's distance learning course, workshops, and seminars held in the United States and Canada are also available.

Earth Garden
Essential Oil and Herbal Dispensary
2, Fairview Parade, Mawney Road, Romford RM7 7HH England
Telephone / Fax 00-44-1708-722633

For a reply and brochure please enclose an International Reply Coupon
available at your post office.

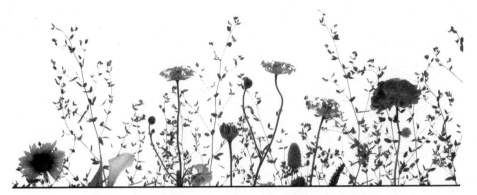

Recommended Reading

If you enjoyed *Aromatherapy for the Healthy Child*, we highly recommend the following books:

The Complete Book of Essential Oils & Aromatherapy by Valerie Ann Worwood. A classic aromatherapy reference, this encyclopedic book contains many health remedies and beauty recipes including sections specifically for women and men, travel, work-related problems, sports, dance, children, the elderly, the home, pets, cooking, gardening, aromatic celebration and treats, and much more.

The Fragrant Mind by Valerie Ann Worwood. A practical encyclopedic book with blends and recipes, concentrating on the emotional, psychological, and mood-changing effects of essential oils. This helpful reference includes A to Z sections on emotional positivity, as well as emotional problems. Worwood also introduces Aroma-Genera, a system of matching personality types with appropriate essential oils.

The Fragrant Heavens by Valerie Ann Worwood. The search for spiritual awareness and enlightenment has become a major force in the modern world as people seek a sense of well-being that goes beyond their need for material things. With *The Fragrant Heavens*, Worwood breaks new ground with her in-depth study of the use of fragrance in spirituality.

Scents & Scentuality by Valerie Ann Worwood. All you need to know about the use of essential oils to enhance sensuality and sexual pleasure.

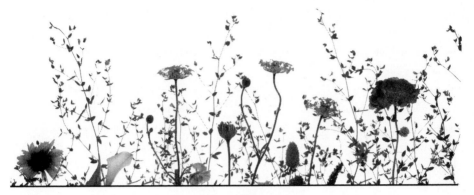

Index

N

O

P

R

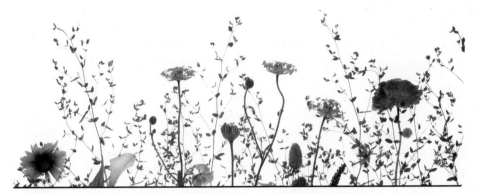

About the Author

Valerie Ann Worwood is internationally acknowledged as one of the world's leading aromatherapists. She is the author of the bestselling *The Complete Book of Essential Oils & Aromatherapy, The Fragrant Mind, The Fragrant Heavens,* and *Scents & Scentuality.* Awarded a doctorate in 1990, she has served on the executive councils of the International Federation of Aromatherapists and the Aromatherapy Organizations Council and has conducted numerous research projects in the clinical use of essential oils. She lives in Essex, England.